UNDERSTANDING ALLERGIES

UNDERSTANDING

ALLERGIES

by

JOHN W. GERRARD, D.M., F.R.C.P.
Professor of Pediatrics
University of Saskatchewan
Saskatoon, Canada

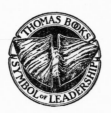

CHARLES C THOMAS • PUBLISHER
Springfield • Illinois • U.S.A.

Published and Distributed Throughout the World by
CHARLES C THOMAS • PUBLISHER
Bannerstone House
301-327 East Lawrence Avenue, Springfield, Illinois, U.S.A.

© *1973, by* CHARLES C THOMAS • PUBLISHER
ISBN 0-398-02768-4

Library of Congress Catalog Card Number: 73-1394

*With THOMAS BOOKS careful attention is given to all details of
manufacturing and design. It is the Publisher's desire to present books
that are satisfactory as to their physical qualities and artistic possibilities
and appropriate for their particular use. THOMAS BOOKS will be true
to those laws of quality that assure a good name and good will.*

Printed in the United States of America

EE-11

TO
Betty,
Jon,
Peter
and
Chris

PREFACE

It is my hope that this little book will provide you, the parents of an allergic child, with background information so that you may better understand the nature of your child's complaint. When an accident or an attack of appendicitis strikes a child, the parents have no alternative but to place him in the hands of a competent physician or surgeon, and leave everything to him. But should the child develop diabetes, for example, the parents must learn all that they can about this disorder, for they themselves have to participate in the child's care and management. In this respect allergies resemble diabetes. The doctor, except in emergencies such as an acute attack of asthma, can do very little by himself, he needs the help of the parents, and if the parents are to help him they must understand.

This little book is not a self-service manual, for your child should be under the care of a doctor, whether a family physician, pediatrician or allergist. It is he who is guiding and helping you, but he may not have time to provide you with all the background information that you need. It is my hope that this book will tell you some of the things that he himself would have told you, had he had the time.

It is possible, possibly probable, that your doctor may not agree with all that I have written. This should surprise neither you nor me. The frontiers of the field of allergy are still ill defined, and the details of many allergic reactions are still far from clear. Some excellent physicians and neurologists consider, for example, that migraine is only exceptionally due to allergy, likewise most physicians believe that enuresis is a developmental disorder. In my own experience allergy often plays a key role in both disorders. Perhaps, when all the facts are known, the truth will be found to lie somewhere in between.

I hope that the illustrations prove helpful. You may be surprised to find so many related to foods. The reasons for this are twofold. First, most of the problems that I encounter are in babies and young children, and in this group of patients foods play a prominent role. Secondly, reactions to foods, when they can be identified, are often more clear cut than are the reactions to inhalants. It is easier, for example, to demonstrate that drinking milk makes a child's nose run than that exposure to house dust does so, even though house dust is probably a much commoner cause of *allergic rhinitis*. The relationship to milk is easier to demonstrate, for the child can be taken off milk and made better, and then put back on milk and made worse. It is not so easy to take him away from house dust, and then to expose him to it.

In conclusion I would like to thank those who have helped me with my studies. First and foremost is the late Dr. Lawson Wilkins, who taught me the importance of a careful, thorough and unhurried history and examination. Second are the family physicians who have kindly presented me with some of their more troublesome problems. Third are the problem children and their parents, from them I have learned more than they realize. And fourth are those who were kind enough to read the manuscript, in part or in whole: Drs. W. G. Crook, W. C. Deamer, J. Glaser, R. N. Hamburger, L. W. Hardy, D. C. Heiner, G. B. Logan, A. Murray, M. K. Shokeir, S. C. Siegel, and F. Speer. I am grateful to them for their comments. I have incorporated many of their suggestions, and if the book is found to be both acceptable and helpful this will be due in no small measure to them. J.W.G.
Saskatoon

CONTENTS

UNDERSTANDING ALLERGIES

Chapter I

THE MANIFESTATIONS OF ALLERGY I

You have been told that your child is allergic. What does this mean? It means that he is reacting abnormally in a special sort of way to something he has touched, smelled, breathed, eaten, or been injected with. Let me give you an example. A number of years ago I went with my family for our summer holiday to the seaside. Our youngest, Chris, was then two months old. He was still being breast fed. One morning he woke with puffy eyelids and large, red raised welts on his body. During the night he had developed urticaria or, as many people would say, hives.

Urticaria is an allergic reaction and nearly always indicates that the individual afflicted has eaten or been exposed to something to which he is allergic. But Chris had had nothing apart from breast milk, and he certainly had not had an injection. We wondered if he could have been upset by some food eaten by my wife, a food to which he and not she, was allergic, traces of which had reached him through the breast. The day before his rash developed, my wife had eaten fresh crab for the first time since his birth. She decided to avoid crab for the time being and the hives disappeared.

Years later Chris ate a smidgeon of crab meat at a party and back came the hives. His attack of hives was an allergic reaction to crab. So when we say that someone is allergic, we mean that he reacts abnormally to or is upset by something that most of us tolerate. This *something* is called an allergen. Foods are just one of many factors that are allergens to some people. We have, for example, a young friend whose eyes and nose run whenever he is near a dog, or even enters a room in which there has been a dog. He is allergic to dog dander. Dog dander, quite harmless to most of us, is an allergen to him.

From these two examples it can be seen that allergic reactions do not always affect the same part of the body. In the first the skin was affected, in the second the eyes and nose. The reactions, however, tend to repeat themselves in the same individual. Chris, if he continues to react to crab, will probably always do so by developing hives. But not everyone who is allergic to crab develops hives or urticaria, nor does everyone who is allergic to dogs develop hay fever.

In fact the dog who is sleeping by the fire may affect the nose of one person, making him sneeze, and the lungs of another, making him wheeze; and when he gets up and rubs a friendly shoulder against another person's legs, he may irritate the skin so that it becomes red and itchy. He may make it, as we say, eczematous. Before we discuss these reactions further, I think we should make quite sure that we know what we mean by terms such as hay fever, eczema, and asthma. We should also know how the allergic reaction affects the different parts of the body.

Hay Fever

Hay fever upsets the normal function of the nose. This is a very important member of the body. It not only warms or cools the air we breathe, it also filters it, removing dust particles, so that when the air enters our lungs, it is relatively clean. Because all air entering the lungs normally passes through the nose, the nose is able to monitor the environment. It tells us that somewhere in the kitchen the gas is leaking, that cakes are burning, or that the roast is ready. For the same reason it is often the first to suffer in the allergic reaction. Pollens from grasses and trees, dusts, and molds, in fact anything in the air, passes through the nose. If the owner of the nose is allergic, the odds are that his nose will begin to itch and then to pour out large quantities of watery mucous.

The conjunctiva, a fine membrane which covers the whites of the eyeballs and the lining of the eyelids, are similarly exposed to particles in the air. When the eyes and nose run and the mucous membrane lining the nose becomes swollen on exposure to an allergen, it is often said that the person has hay fever; allergists usually call it *allergic rhinitis.* The swelling of the nasal mucosa tends to block the little openings into the sinuses and also the narrow tube, the *Eustachian Tube,* which leads to the *middle ear.* The ears are connected to the outside world through this *Eustachian Tube.* The *middle ear* normally contains air, that is why ears tend to pop when outside pressures change rapidly when we are in an airplane. If the openings into the ears and sinuses become blocked, the fluid which forms cannot get out and the ears and sinuses become inflamed. If the blockage of the *Eustachian Tube* persists, the person may become temporarily or even permanently deaf.

Asthma

In asthma the lungs and bronchial tubes are affected by the allergic reaction. These, like the nose, seem to be very vulnerable to allergens, particularly to those in the air such as pollens and house dust. Just as the mucous membranes of the nose become swollen and secrete watery mucous in hay fever, so, in asthma, the linings of the bronchial tubes are irritated and become swollen. Again clear, sticky mucous is secreted. The asthmatic's breathing becomes noisy, and he develops a rattle in his chest and a troublesome cough.

Added to the above, the smooth muscle in the wall of the bronchial tubes contracts so that the tubes become narrow, and the patient has increasing difficulty in breathing. He usually finds it more difficult to breathe out than to breathe in, and when he breathes out, he wheezes. If his tubes or chest become very tight, he may find himself fighting for breath. His lungs may even become over distended with air which he has inspired but which he cannot completely expire; blood is deprived of oxygen which it needs and, in some severe cases, carbon dioxide, a waste product which is normally disposed of in the breath, accumulates in the blood.

Urticaria

As we have already mentioned, the skin also may be affected by allergens. People who live in parts of the world where stinging nettles grow know that where they are stung the skin becomes itchy and swollen. The center of the swollen area is usually pale, the edges usually pink. The swelling is due to the liberation of a chemical called histamine. Urticaria or hives, though often more extensive, has an identical appearance. It, too, is due to the liberation of histamine. Urticarial lesions tend to come and go. They can occur on any part of the body. They are not usually dangerous, but if the swelling happens to involve the throat and windpipe, it may cause asphyxia and death.

Sometimes the cause of the urticaria is self-evident, as it was in the case of Chris. Sometimes it is not, and it may never be known what caused it. Luckily, in its milder form, urticaria never causes permanent disability. Antihistamines usually control it, and no harm comes from not knowing what has caused it.

Eczema

Eczema, or *atopic dermatitis,* exists in two main forms. The first is more commonly seen in babies. It usually starts when the baby is only a few weeks or months old, often as a redness on the cheeks, chin, and forehead. It may spread to cover the whole of the body or, in less severe cases, just to the creases behind the knees and in front of the elbows and wrists. The rash is extraordinarily itchy. The baby, if given half a chance, will rub the skin raw and may even make it bleed. This form of the rash seems to have been much more troublesome when babies were brought up on ordinary cow's milk, before the advent of the modern prepared canned formulas.

The rash is sometimes caused by foods, and if, for example, it is due to cow's milk and only to cow's milk, it will clear up completely when the baby is taken off cow's milk. It may also be due to contact with fur, wool, baby oils, soaps, and so on. I remember one baby who was admitted to the hospital with very extensive eczema. His skin became normal, helped no doubt by the treatment that we gave him. When his mother came to fetch him, his skin was as smooth as the skin of a new born baby. But by the time she had carried him to the front door of the hospital, contact with her fur coat—she had cuddled him close since it was very cold outside—had brought out the rash all over his face.

Once the cause is known, eczema can be cured quickly simply by taking the baby off the food (s) or by keeping him away from the soap or wool to which he is allergic. If its cause remains undiscovered, and this is sometimes the case, it may persist for a number of years, though its severity can nearly always be greatly reduced by the application of lotions or ointments. It is, however, wise to try to find out the cause of the eczema since babies with eczema sometimes develop asthma as they grow older. Whatever has caused the eczema may also play a part in causing the asthma. Asthma may be a much more serious and troublesome problem, and only when we know exactly what is causing it can we help to prevent the occurrence of further attacks.

The second form of eczema is usually called *contact dermatitis*. This, as its name implies, is a red irritation of the skin which develops where it has been in contact with something to which the patient is allergic. Nickel rings, zippers and other objects made with nickel, ointments, hair dyes, and dyes in clothes can all cause this type of eczema, and because it is usually well localized, it is generally not too difficult to determine its cause.

Vomiting, Diarrhea, Colic, and Constipation

Doctors who look after babies, and mothers too, know that some babies are upset by their formulas; some, but not all, of these reactions may be allergic. A number of years ago a friend of mine was asked to see a nine-month-old child who was extraordinarily allergic to cow's milk. This baby was still on the breast. His mother was finding it difficult to wean him off the breast, because every time she gave him cow's milk, he threw it all back. He had never vomited breast milk. He vomited cow's milk because he was allergic to it, and wherever the milk landed on his skin, he blistered. This reaction was so violent and so clearly related to cow's milk that no one had any hesitation in saying that he was allergic to cow's milk.

A few years later I was asked to see a six-week-old baby girl who had had diarrhea since birth. Whatever the formula, cow's milk, goat's milk, soya milk, the diarrhea persisted. Luckily breast milk was available in a local breast milk bank and on this her diarrhea stopped. We were able to test her reactions to a variety of foods and eventually found a few she tolerated. This little baby was allergic to many foods.

Allergic reactions which involve the bowel usually cause vomiting, diarrhea, or both. Occasionally they cause constipation. Babies developing constipation may have normal, soft bowel movements when on their ordinary formula, even though it is made from cow's milk, or on the breast, but when given ordinary cow's milk, boiled or unboiled, promptly become constipated. I have seen one family in which everyone except the father had to avoid cow's milk because it made them all constipated. We are not sure that this reaction is truly an allergic one, but it may be; it certainly is an abnormal reaction to something which does not upset most of us.

With regard to colic, babies with allergies have more than their fair share of colic, and colic is sometimes an allergic problem, but I am not sure that it always is. Some babies seem to be colicky whatever they are given, though others stop crying and squirming when they are taken off cow's milk. I encourage a mother with a colicky baby to try to find a formula or food that suits him. If she cannot, I advise her to wait patiently until her baby *grows out of it.* This is easier said than done.

Chapter II

THE MANIFESTATIONS OF ALLERGY II

Bed-wetting or Nocturnal Enuresis

All normal babies are wet, almost constantly. It is only when they are a year or two old that they begin to develop adequate control of their bladders and become dry. By the age of four most normal children are consistently dry. So that it is only when a child is four or over that we begin to be concerned about bed-wetting. There are many obvious reasons why some children wet the bed at night. Some lack normal control of the bladder because the nervous supply is defective; this happens in children whose spinal cords have not developed normally. Some children with sugar diabetes wet the bed at night because they pass large amounts of watery urine; they lose weight in spite of good appetites. Some children with bladder infections wet the bed at night, others do so simply because they drink too much before going to bed.

Bed-wetting may also occur if the child is very tired and sleeps heavily. In most instances, however, the child who wets the bed does so for no very obvious reason. His urine and bladder are normal; the nerve supply is intact. He himself is bright and obedient, doing reasonably well at school. His parents are kind and considerate, and the home has no more problems than any other normal home—save that Tommy, or less commonly Jane, wets the bed, sometimes every night, sometimes only once or twice a week. Why he is sometimes dry and sometimes wet, no one really seems to know.

Just over forty years ago a Dr. Bray, an Australian physician who had settled in London and who had made a special study of allergic problems in children, noticed that several of his allergic patients, when cured of their asthma, unexpectedly became dry

9

at night. One of his patients was a boy of five who had always wet the bed. He came to see Dr. Bray because, for three months, he had had severe attacks of asthma which were always preceded by intense stomach aches and were accompanied by more frequent lapses of enuresis. In spite of fluid restrictions, the administration of belladonna, and waking him up at night, the enuresis continued unabated.

Skin tests were positive to wheat. Wheat was excluded from his diet. For the next eighteen months, while he remained on a wheat-free diet, he suffered from neither enuresis nor asthma. Another patient was a three-year-old boy who suffered from eczema, asthma, and enuresis. His skin tests were positive to feathers, horse hair, egg, pork, potato, and rice. These were removed from his environment or diet, and he had no further attacks of asthma and was dry at night.

The asthma and eczema experienced by the above children were certainly allergic reactions; we suspect that the bed-wetting also was. Other allergists have observed enuresis in association with allergies, and so have we, but the truth of the matter is that most enuretics do not have obvious allergies. When this is the case, why are they enuretic?

Several groups of doctors in the United States, Canada, and Sweden have studied the sizes of the bladders of bed-wetting and normal children and have found that the bladders of most bed-wetting children are small. Studies to determine the size of the child's bladder are usually carried out in one of two ways. First, the child may be given a pint of water to drink and then asked to refrain from passing urine for as long as possible. The amount of urine passed when he is about to burst is measured, as is the next volume; the larger of these two volumes indicates the maximum size of his bladder.

Secondly, the parents may be asked to measure and record for a whole week the amounts of urine that their bed-wetting and non-bed-wetting children pass. The largest volume that any one child passes indicates the maximum size of his bladder. It is nearly always found that the bed-wetting child, taking his age into consideration, has a much smaller bladder capacity than has his normal brother or sister, and that during the daytime he passes smaller amounts of urine more frequently than his dry brother or sister does.

Studies such as these have shown that most enuretics, at least three-quarters, have small bladders, and they pass urine frequently during the daytime, as well as wet the bed at night. The children with the smallest bladders wet themselves not only during the night, but also during the daytime. They are, according to their mothers, *always wet*. They are often thought to be lazy and are frequently scolded on this account. In point of fact they are not lazy; they have such small, irritable bladders that they cannot get to the toilet in time, and it is for this reason that they are always wet.

At one time it was thought that the enuretic's bladder was made small, as though he had been given a size two bladder for a size four body. At one time I agreed with this concept, but I can no longer do so for studies carried out with colleagues have made it seem that the bladder of the enuretic is small because it is in spasm; just as the bronchial tubes of the asthmatic are small because they too are in spasm. If this is the explanation, we would expect the enuretic children to be allergic. I had not read Dr. Bray's studies at this time, and previously, when asked to see an enuretic child, I would simply make certain that he had no demonstrable disease and would then give him a *placebo*, a harmless drug, assuring him at the same time that if he were to take it regularly at night, it would cure his enuresis, and sometimes it did.

One spring a few years ago, I was asked to see a child who was wetting the bed nightly. She was a perfectly normal child, and to my delight she responded to treatment with a placebo and became dry all through the summer. Unfortunately she started to wet the bed again as soon as the fall term started. She remained wet all through the winter but became dry once more in the summer, only to become wet again when the fall term started. She was a bright, intelligent girl. She was very distressed by her disability and at night would stay awake, sometimes for hours, trotting to and fro from the toilet to make sure that her bladder was empty when at last she fell asleep. She would nevertheless be wet again when she woke in the morning.

Her bed-wetting was linked so clearly with school that we felt that even though she said that she loved school she probably had a hidden reason for not liking it. But on close questioning it transpired, and why I do not know, that in the summer she preferred to drink juices and Kool-Aids only; while in the winter, as soon as school started, she preferred milk. We asked her to stop drinking milk and she promptly became dry. It was the milk and not the school that made her enuretic.

A little later I saw another child who wet the bed regularly at home but who was always dry when on holiday at the lake. At home she drank much milk; at the lake, as the family did not have a refrigerator at their cottage, she drank only juices. Again, it was the milk which was making her wet the bed, and when she stopped drinking milk at home, she remained dry.

From all the above I think we may conclude that the normal functioning of the nose and lungs, of the stomach and intestines, and of the bladder can be disturbed by the allergic process. Inhalants and foods that do not upset most of us can, in the allergic individual, make his nose run, his bronchial tubes contract, his stomach vomit, his bowel hurry on its contents, or make his bladder contract so that he has to pass urine frequently; if he is a child, he will probably wet the bed at night.

It is natural at this juncture to ask ourselves why these parts of the body should be singled out. Is it also possible that other parts of the body could be similarly affected? The first question will remain unanswered for the time being. The second can be answered in the affirmative; there are other tissues affected by the allergic process and they are the blood vessels.

The Vascular System

The blood vessels are involved in three separate situations. The very small vessels or capillaries are involved in urticaria; we have discussed this condition briefly already. Urticarial lesions are always raised above the level of the skin because the capillaries become dilated and allow fluids to leak out into the tissue spaces. The larger blood vessels or arteries are affected in migraine. The blood vessels involved are usually those supplying the head, and this includes the brain as well as the superficial tissues such as the face and scalp. Usually only a few blood vessels are involved in any one attack. The same blood vessels are probably involved in subsequent attacks, and when this is so, each attack is a repeat performance.

At the onset of the attack, the affected blood vessels become narrow. If the vessels are superficial, the face will become pale; if the vessels are deep inside the skull, the supply of glucose and oxygen to the brain will be reduced. Brain function may be interfered with. If the vessels over the back of the brain in the occipital area (this is concerned with vision) are narrowed, the patient's vision may be disturbed, objects may become suddenly blurred, or segments of his field of vision may be lost, and he is temporarily blind. In the area in which he is for the time being blind, bright flashing lights, like the edges of a saw, or flashes of lightning may appear.

If vessels supplying other parts of the brain are involved, there may be a temporary disturbance of sensation such as tingling or dizziness or even weakness leading to paralysis. These warning signs normally last a minute or two, but they may persist for as long as 20 to 30 minutes. As they subside, they are replaced, in a classical attack, by a throbbing headache. This sensation is sometimes generalized, as though the whole head was *splitting;* sometimes it is localized, for example, to one side of the head. It may even be localized to a discrete spot, often in the region of the temple.

When describing his headache, the sufferer may put his finger on the spot and say that this is where his head hurts. The pain may be so acute that the child with migraine may cry. During an attack he usually likes to lie curled up undisturbed in the dark. If he manages to fall asleep, he will wake up an hour or two later fully restored and refreshed. Not all migraine headaches follow this classical progression; some headaches are constant, and the sufferer has to learn to *live with them.*

Migraine headaches are often associated, particularly in children, with nausea and vomiting. The child may not recover until he has vomited his heart out. Following this he will probably fall asleep. When he wakes up, he will probably be *raring to go*. When migraine is associated with vomiting, it is often called a *bilious attack*.

The adult with this syndrome is very much aware of the sequence of events: the disturbance of vision, followed by a throbbing, unbearable headache, and repeated spells of vomiting. The child who has migraine, and many children do, cannot usually describe his attacks in the same detail, and though he will probably point a finger to his head and sometimes to one particular spot saying *head hurts*, he may simply turn pale, be obviously unwell, go to bed, and proceed to vomit. In severe cases the child may continue to vomit until he has been given an intravenous infusion of glucose, and only then will his vomiting cease. In milder instances he may only have twinges of pain in his abdomen, and when this is the case, he will probably say *my tummy hurts*. Children who have spells of tummy pain frequently develop classical migraine after puberty.

Not all doctors who treat children are aware of this because most of their patients grow out of their age range, but on the staff of one of Canada's most famous children's hospitals, there are a group of pediatricians who themselves experienced this sequence of events and who are for personal reasons very much aware of the relationship. The clinical picture of vomiting without conspicuous headache is not uncommon in children and is often called the *recurrent abdominal pain syndrome, periodic disorder* or *cyclical vomiting*, or even *abdominal migraine*.

A third situation in which the vascular system is involved in the *allergic* process is in a catastrophic reaction called anaphylaxis. We will defer discussion of this until later.

Allergic Reactions Involving the Nervous System

A few years ago I was trying to find out how common unsuspected allergies were. I did this by looking for allergic problems in children being seen for other reasons, for example, a heart murmur or convulsions. One such child, being treated for epilepsy, tended to have frequent colds. Frequent colds are often a manifestation of an *allergic rhinitis*. Allergic rhinitis is usually due to inhalants such as house dust, but sometimes it is due to foods, such as milk. This child was drinking much milk, so I asked his mother to keep him off milk and dairy products for a month and to let me know whether his nose stopped runing; if it did, she was once more to give him milk to see if his *cold* returned. Six weeks later she telephoned to say that her son's nose had indeed dried up, but she had decided not to place him back on milk because milk had had such a disturbing effect on his personality.

"How come?" I asked. She went on to explain that her son, Charles, used to be a restless, inattentive lad who was so fidgety in the classroom that he infuriated his teacher and upset most of the other children. About ten days after he had stopped drinking milk, his teacher had dropped into their home to ask if Charles' medicine had been increased. The teacher knew that he had been to the hospital for his annual checkup. "No," said his mother, "why do you ask?"

"Well," replied his teacher, "something has happened to him. He used to be restless, fidgety, and inattentive. Since going to the hospital, he has become as good as gold. He now concentrates on his work, he sits as still as a statue, and is a model to everyone else." His mother did not want to give him milk because she was certain that it was the milk which had made him such a trial for his teacher.

More recently I was asked to see a child with a bed-wetting problem who had also been driving his parents crazy because he was always on the go; he never gave them a moment's peace. His parents did not mention his disposition when we discussed his enuresis. After the preliminary studies had been completed, I asked his mother to take him off certain foods, these included milk and dairy products, and to report back in three weeks time. When she returned, I asked if he was dry at night. "No," she replied, "he is wetting the bed as often as ever, but he is a different boy."

"Can you explain?" I asked. In reply she went on to say that when she had taken Tim, her son, home, her husband had naturally wanted to know how we were hoping to cure his enuresis.

When he had learned that we were only asking Tim to stop drinking milk and a few other foods and that we were not even giving him any medicine, he was immediately hostile. He was at first unwilling, but later reluctantly agreed, to let Tim be placed on the restricted diet and to be kept on it for two weeks. As soon as the two weeks were over, he gave Tim a glass of milk to drink and an hour later a second glass. Tim promptly became *a ball of fire*. He went wild and was quite uncontrollable. His parents previously had not realized that his *character* had changed on his restricted diet, but the prompt return of his wild behavior when he drank a glass of milk left them in no doubt that drinking milk changed his whole personality. "He must never have another glass," his father declared.

At first I found it hard to believe that harmless foods could so change a child's personality; but many parents have made confirmatory, unsolicited observations, and I am now fully convinced that in ways we do not yet understand, the allergic child's, and adult's too, behavior can be altered and modified as dramatically by foods as it can be altered by drugs. The following examples indicate the bizarre nature of these problems. A medical student who had hay fever, and who has had many attacks of asthma, has to avoid foods containing corn because corn makes him feel so drowsy that he can hardly keep his eyes open.

An internist has found that he has to avoid foods containing egg and wheat because these two foods make him irritable and irascible. His wife, who now naturally prepares his food with great care, finds him at such times impossible to live with. Two pediatric acquaintances both find that coffee, which keeps most people awake, puts them to sleep; one, if he has difficulty in getting to sleep at night, gets up and brews himself a strong cup of coffee and then sleeps as sounds as a bell. Quite the opposite sometimes happens when certain children are given phenobarbitone. Phenobarbitone makes most people sleepy, but it makes some children so irritable and cantankerous that they drive their parents *up the wall*. We have still much to learn about these unnatural reactions to foods and drugs. They are probably the cause of the rather tense, restless, and even unreasonable behavior exhibited by some allergic individuals.

Those allergists who have made a special study of children who are sometimes tense and sometimes unaccountably tired, say that these children have, in the words of Dr. Speer, the *Tension Fatigue Syndrome*. As a florid example of this disorder I can do no better than quote the observations of a very perceptive mother. "My nine year old daughter, Sarah," she said, "behaves normally on a restricted diet, but within a few hours of eating a bar of chocolate will have a nose bleed, and will have repeated nose bleeds for the next few days. She will fly angrily at her younger brother who teases her slightly. On being asked to lay the table or to pick up something from the floor she will break into tears and run to her room. In the evening she will complain of being unable to sleep, and will be afraid of having a nightmare. She will wet the bed in the middle of the night and then wake up. In the morning, having had a bad night's sleep, she will be dazed and have dark circles under her eyes. She will hardly be able to get herself together to get off to school. Her appetite will be poor, though she will crave sweets and pickles. She will come home after school with a story of not feeling well in school and of not getting along with the other children. Her teacher will say that she has been unhappy, fidgety and inattentive, and that her performance in mathematics and spelling has been deficient. The troubles of the previous night will repeat themselves. She may also have other complaints such as an itchy *bottom,* a stomach ache or headache. The restlessness will taper off during the course of the next day, and then she will be back to normal."

Chapter III

COMMON ALLERGENS I

In the last chapter we discussed the parts of the body commonly involved in the allergic reaction. In this chapter we will talk about the allergens and irritants, those things that start off or trigger the allergic response. They include the following:

1. INHALANTS. Substances that are breathed in. These include house dust, pollens from trees, grasses, and weeds, and emanations from feathers and animal fur. They also include perfumes, aromas from paints and foods, insecticides, tobacco smoke, gasses, and smog. In fact anything in the air which has been known to cause asthma or hay fever or other allergic reactions. These particles or aromas are caught up in the nose or penetrate the lungs. They may also be absorbed through the bowel if spit containing them is swallowed.

2. INGESTANTS. Substances that are eaten or swallowed. These include all foods and food additives, as well as drugs that are taken by mouth or given by suppository.

3. INJECTANTS. Substances that are injected. These include antibiotics injected on purpose, such as penicillin, and bee, wasp, and other strings injected on purpose by the insect but not by the recipient.

4. CONTACTANTS. Substances with which the body is in contact. These include things which we touch by choice: wool, silk, clothes of all kinds, dyes, soaps, creams, detergents, jewelry, zippers, etc., as well as things that we touch inadvertently, such as poison ivy.

5. INFECTIONS. Infections, particularly of the lungs in children, often precipitate attacks of asthma. This happens so frequently that some children appear to be allergic to whatever germ is causing the infection. This may sometimes be the case, though more frequently the infection probably brings to light or aggravates an underlying allergy.

6. Physical factors: such as exposure to cold and exercise and psychological factors should also be considered, although they may not be allergens in the strict use of the term.

As the reader must now realize, there is an almost limitless number of substances to which people can be, and some are, allergic. When it is also appreciated that most allergic individuals are sensitive to more than one allergen, it becomes apparent that unravelling allergic problems is not always straightforward. And yet if we are to help your allergic child with his problems, we must first find out what he is allergic to, for only by so doing can we help him to avoid it; this is the most effective form of treatment. Prevention in the field of allergy is always better than cure. The alternatives are to arrange for a course of *shots* if the allergen is an inhalant and cannot be avoided or to treat him symptomatically by giving him an antihistamine or other suitable medicine, and in this way to relieve his symptoms as best we can.

How are we going to find out what he is allergic to? This only can be done effectively if you and your doctor cooperate; you have to be a Dr. Watson and he a Sherlock Holmes. In this search the most vital information is the history; this provides the clues and the circumstantial evidence necessary to identify the culprit or culprits. The tests which your doctor will order do not provide a short cut. They serve another purpose. The x-rays, blood, urine, nasal and skin tests are carried out first to ensure that your child does not have a disease that behaves like an allergy but isn't, and then to provide confirmatory evidence that he does in fact have an allergic problem. In exceptional circumstances, when the history provides a dearth of clues, greater weight may need to be placed on the tests.

Inhalants

Pollen. What would lead you to suspect that inhalants are to blame? First that the child's symptoms are seasonal. Pollen grains are the plant counterpart to human sperm. Somehow or other the pollen has to reach the female *egg* housed in the *stigma* of the flower. Plants with beautiful blooms and attractive scents are usually pollinated by bees, butterflies, and hummingbirds. As a reward for their labors the flowers usually provide them with nectar. The pollen from these flowers tends to be heavy and sticky, and because it is carried from flower to flower, it does not cause much hay fever or asthma.

Most plants, however, depend on the wind for cross pollination. These plants of necessity have to produce literally clouds of pollen, for they have to almost saturate the air with pollen if the pollen is going to reach, in an entirely random fashion, at least a few of the flowers waiting to be pollinated. These are the pollen grains that cause most trouble. The flowers pollinated in this way are, for the most part, dull and drab.

To increase the chances of pollination, deciduous trees usually make their pollen early in the season before the leaves can shield the flowers. Pollen from trees, therefore, usually causes trouble early in spring, February, March, April, and May in the South and in April, May, and June in the North. Pollens from grasses take to the air a little later in May, June, and July. The grasses most likely to cause trouble are those growing on the lawns and in the fields around your home. Later in the season, from August to September, come the weeds, and of these, ragweed in the East is by far and away the most troublesome; sage and Russian thistle, tumbleweed, tend to cause more trouble on the prairies and in the West. If your newspaper gives the daily pollen counts for your area, you may be able to guess, if your child has hay fever or asthma due to pollen, which type of pollen grain is causing his trouble.

MOLDS. Molds are present in virtually all soils and also in damp and musty homes. Basements are sometimes damp when all other rooms in the house are dry. Molds also grow on foods, are present in cheeses, and have contaminated air conditioners in homes and cars, and humidifiers, leading to outbreaks of asthma, for example, in a secretarial staff. Musty places are usually moldy. Molds in the home are present all the year round; molds in the air outside are most numerous in summer and fall, though in warm climates they are present the year round. Allergies in colder climates due to molds tend to come to a sudden halt with freeze-up or with the first snow.

Trouble from thaw to freeze-up? Think of molds. This aphorism does not apply to the South, for there molds cause trouble the year round. The problems that may arise are well illustrated by the experience of a doctor who moved from a dry area in Southern California, thirty miles from the coast, to a relatively damp one, a mile from the ocean, where he was blanketed by fog for two months out of the twelve. Soon after moving into his new home, he developed asthma which worsened whenever he entered his home from outside and whenever he read books pulled down from his shelves. He was allergic to molds and found himself trapped in a moldy house.

He tried to get rid of the molds with chemicals, only to find that he became allergic to the chemicals. He then tried *shots*, but he was so sensitive to the molds that the shots, even though they were exceedingly weak, made him ill. He had no alternative but to get rid of the molds or abandon his home. He decided to try to get rid of the molds by drying his house out. He bought a *dehumidifier*. The dehumidifier removed up to 18 pints of muddy water daily from the air. The mold count fell. His home no longer smelled musty. He could breathe once more, and though his asthma did not disappear completely, it was controllable; and strange to say, when the molds in his house had been reduced, he was able to take *shots* without being made ill. He was then desensitized.

HOUSE DUST. House dust contains many potential allergens: dust from cushions, furniture, pillows and mattresses, and mold spores and pollens brought in from outside. It may also contain dander from horses, cattle, and other farm animals, as well as grain dust if the father has been in contact with these. It may also contain perfumes and sprays if the mother uses them.

In addition, it will almost certainly contain many tiny mites. This tiny mite was recently identified by a group of Dutch workers. It is so small that it cannot be spotted by the naked eye; 800 lined up shoulder to shoulder would form a line only an inch long. It lives happily on scales of human skin. As the average man or woman sheds two to five pounds of scales a year, the mite has made his home in our homes. He is thoroughly domesticated. He is found in almost every sample of house dust, but his *castle,* his home of election, seems to be the mattress. Here he finds scales of human skin in abundance, and here he is least likely to be swept off his feet by his arch enemy, the vacuum. From the allergist's point of view there appear to be two important mites, *Dermatophagoides pteronyssinus,* the commoner, and *Dermatophagoides farinae.*

People who are allergic to house dust tend to develop symptoms maximally in the winter, at least in the northern climates; for in winter the children play inside rather than outside, and the furnace keeps the dust, which has lain dormant in the vents all summer, in perpetual motion. Children and adults who are allergic to house dust tend to wake up in the morning with stuffy noses, sticky eyes, and loose coughs due to phlegm in their throats and no wonder, they may have slept all night on a mattress full of mites.

If your child, or anyone in your house, is allergic to house dust, it is vitally important to rid the house of as much dust as possible. Special attention should be given to the bedroom because this is the mite's castle and because this is where your child spends most of his time. It is not my intention to write a manual on the treatment and management of asthma, but house dust control is so important that if you have an asthmatic child in your family, you should ideally do the following:

1. Strip the bedroom to its bare minimum. Remove carpets and anything on which dust can settle. Simple cotton or plastic curtains are preferable to venetian blinds.

2. The floor should be damp mopped at first and vacuumed daily.

3. The mattress should be sealed in a nonallergenic zippered cover. Foam rubber pillows and mattresses should be avoided; they tend to harbor molds. Dacron pillows are good.

4. The sheets should be made of cotton and the blankets of synthetic material. Wool, feathers, comforters stuffed with kapok or cotton linters should be avoided.

5. No animals or stuffed toys should be allowed into or kept in the room.

6. The rest of the house should be kept as dust free as possible,

special attention being paid to the heater and its filters.

7. Smoking. Ideally no one in the house should smoke. Those who presently do so should stop, both for their own health's sake but more especially, for their child's.

Foods

As we have already mentioned, some people react so briskly and so strikingly to a given food that they are obviously allergic to it. The baby who vomited cow's milk and whose skin blistered when the milk fell on his skin was such a baby. Even the originator of *every body needs milk* would have agreed that that baby did not. The individual who reacts violently to a food almost invariably knows he is allergic to the food in question. But this same individual may be allergic to other foods and be quite unaware of it.

On one occasion we admitted to the hospital a little boy of fifteen months who was anemic. He had been anemic before and had had to have several courses of iron. His hemoglobin had risen while he was receiving iron, but it fell as soon as the iron was stopped. This made us suspect that he might be losing blood. A relatively common and frequently overlooked cause of blood loss in little children is *milk allergy*. Cow's milk under these circumstances seems to irritate the bowel. Each day traces of blood, too small usually to be seen by the eye, are lost from the body. We studied this child's stools for weekly periods when he was given cow's milk and when he was not. Fortunately for us, his mother insisted on spending the days in the hospital, just to keep an eye on us, the doctors. She noticed that when her child was not given milk, his stools became solid and his nose stopped running; and when he was once more given milk, his stools became loose and frequent, and back would come his cold. He was obviously mildly allergic to milk, and it was his mother who really spotted this.

Now we knew, but his mother did not, that milk allergies tend to run in families. So we turned our attention to the rest of the family. There were four other children, two had never been ill, two had been in and out of the hospital all their short lives, one with repeated attacks of pneumonia and the other with asthma. The mother herself had a constant cough, a smoker's cough she told us, but as well as smoking 20 cigarettes a day, she drank a quart of milk. To cut a long story short, the mother and three of her five children were allergic to cow's milk. When they stopped drinking cow's milk, they all lost their coughs, bronchitis, pneumonias, and asthma, and our little patient lost his anemia. When they drank milk, back came all their problems. That these three children and their mother were all allergic to cow's milk, had never been suspected. In fact the mother had originally said, "I can't be allergic to cow's milk; I love it." Some people only suspect food allergies if the bowel is upset or if the patient develops hives, but food allergies can cause asthma without disturbing the normal working of other systems.

The dramatic reactions to food, as we have already noted, are nearly always easily identified, and the foods which cause such troubles, fish, nuts, etc., can usually be easily avoided. The hidden, unsuspected reactions to foods are less easily identified, but the following will help you to decide whether foods may or may not be causing trouble.

1. If the child is seen in infancy, it is usually possible to correlate the development of symptoms with a change in diet, as happened with a doctor's child who was brought to me. This child first began to wheeze when she was five months old. The family lived in a relatively dust free home, but for lack of anything better to do, we tried to get rid of what little dust there was. The wheezing persisted. Not knowing what to suggest, I sat down with the mother and carefully went over the baby's past history. One week before the wheezing had started, the baby had come off the breast, and a cow's milk formula had been substituted. This suggested that cow's milk might be to blame. We took the baby off cow's milk. Her asthma promptly stopped.

Her father, one of our own graduates who had been taught at a time when we did not realize that cow's milk could do this, was reluctant to admit that cow's milk could make his daughter wheeze; so for awhile he kept giving his baby cow's milk, but every time he did so, she wheezed. Two years later the telephone rang to tell me that another baby had been born into the family. She too had begun to wheeze when she came off the breast and went onto cow's milk. Her mother and father were not disturbed; they now knew how to handle her.

The two children in this family had been troubled with wheezing. Another child, Jane, was brought to me at the age of 13 months because she had had a *cold* all her life. Mucous poured constantly from her nose. She had had this, her mother said, ever since she was born. She first caught the cold in the nursery; at this time she was on a cow's milk formula and nothing else. Within a few days of taking her off cow's milk and dairy products, her *cold* went, only to return when she was once more given cow's milk. Not only cow's milk, but any food the child is allergic to can cause troubles of this kind. I have even seen it due to cod liver oil.

2. A food allergy should be suspected in an older child if there is a history of the child's having had food allergies in infancy. If, for example, he had, when small, developed a rash on the face every time he had oranges, his current trouble with asthma, headaches, or recurrent spells of pain may be aggravated or precipitated by the oranges which gave him a rash when he was a baby.

3. If there is a proven or known food allergy in another member of the family, the same food may be causing trouble in this child. One of my colleagues has four children who develop winter colds, bronchitis, or asthma when they drink milk. Only one child in the family, the oldest, seemed to be free from allergies. But though she had no obvious allergies, she began one day to complain of *tummy pains*. No cause could be found for these. It was therefore felt that they too might be due to an allergy. She was taken off milk. The pains vanished. She was given milk. The pains returned. I have been surprised how often the same food causes problems in more than one member of a family.

4. The child who gets recurrent chest colds, repeated attacks of pneumonia, or periodic spells of abdominal pain or vomiting is often allergic to a food which he is taking every day. It is as though by taking the food every day he gradually builds up trouble which breaks out in a bout of pneumonia or in a bilious attack. Following this his system is, as we say, refractory to the

food for two to four weeks, when symptoms return once more. This freedom from trouble is seen quite commonly in animals after an anaphyllactic or severe, allergic reaction.

5. Although foods taken regularly throughout the year would be expected to cause symptoms of equal severity all through the year, this is not always the case. Some children allergic to one or more foods may be able to tolerate these foods in the summer, but if they are also sensitive to house dust, they cannot tolerate them in the winter when they are confined for much of the time to their own dusty homes. If they are taken off the foods they are allergic to in the winter, they are no longer upset by the house dust. Children allergic both to a food and to ragweed may be able to tolerate the food before and after, but not during, the ragweed season. It is as though the child could tolerate either the food in moderation or house dust in moderation, but together they make him wheeze.

In either case the child is helped both by the elimination of the food and by an antidust program. If the doctor who recommended the former is interested in food allergy, he may tell you that this proves that your child is allergic to the food; if the doctor is more concerned with environmental control, he may confidently tell you that your child has grown out of his food allergy and has now acquired a dust allergy.

6. Children, and adults also, are often allergic to the foods which they seem to crave and which they most readily eat. Allergy, like life, is full of paradoxes, and though, as we shall mention later, some children seem to instinctively dislike the food to which they are allergic, and on this account try to avoid it and so remain well; others seem to crave the food they should avoid. I once had a secretary who was often incapacitated by migraine. She kept in her desk a supply of licorice, and she herself seemed to live on licorice. When she realized that some individuals were allergic to the foods on which they depended, she stopped taking licorice and remained free from migraine till one day she nibbled a little just to find out if it really did provoke an attack. She had to take two days off her headache was so severe.

An acquaintance of mine, the father is a doctor, had a son who was troubled with frequent bouts of abdominal pain. Investigations revealed no apparent cause. One day his mother noticed, when he came running to her complaining that his tummy hurt, that her son was chewing gum. She watched him carefully and noted that every time he chewed gum he complained of pain. She took his gum away from him. He remained well. Some weeks later she gave him some gum. Twenty minutes later, she timed it with her watch, the pain returned.

I think it is probable that such children, being fundamentally allergic, become allergic to the food or foods to which they are very frequently exposed, but it is also possible that such children crave the food because they are allergic to it. It may meet some unmet need of the body. I can perhaps best explain this by an illustration.

The father of one our patients had, when we first saw him, a chronic bronchitis; he had had it as long as he could remember. He had been brought up on a farm where milk was always available. He drank on average a litre a day. I first met him after I had seen his baby. His baby had had to be admitted to hospital with a severe bronchopneumonia. When I found out that the baby developed bronchopneumonia if we gave him cow's milk, I asked his father if he would be kind enough to stop drinking cow's milk and taking dairy products to see if he, too, was allergic to milk. He kindly agreed to do this, although he said it would be a hardship for he loved milk. To his surprise his chest cleared completely and his cough vanished.

Three weeks later he came home with some cottage cheese and said to his wife that he had to have it for supper. That night he was in trouble, coughing as much as he had ever coughed before. He discovered later that he could no longer take any milk without becoming incapacitated. When he had been drinking much milk each day, his general health had been excellent, in spite of his cough. When he had stopped drinking milk, he found that even traces incapacitated him.

This is not an isolated illustration; so I think that it is possible that in ways that we do not yet understand, the craving for a food to which an individual is allergic may help him to tolerate it, at least to some degree. It is paradoxes such as these which make it difficult for us to lay down hard and fast rules about the management of food allergies.

Chapter IV

COMMON ALLERGENS II

Substances That Are Injected

When we discussed the common manifestations of allergy, asthma, hay fever, hives, etc., we omitted mentioning anaphylaxis. This is the word used to describe the most sudden and catastrophic of all the allergic reactions. The term was coined at the turn of the century by two French doctors who were studying the mechanism of immunity.

Many children now growing up will never develop diphtheria, poliomyelitis, or tetanus. This is because they have been immunized *prophylactically* by being given shots either by needle or sometimes, as in the case of polio, by mouth. Generally speaking, children react most vigorously to the first of such a series of shots and, because they then build up an immunity, less to subsequent injections. This is illustrated best by the reaction to smallpox vaccination. Ten to twelve days after the first vaccination the child normally develops a swollen arm, an angry little ulcer surrounded by an area of inflammation, and a fever. After a second vaccination the child will probably develop no more than a small, itchy, pink lesion about an eighth of an inch in diameter.

This is what the French doctors expected when they immunized their dogs. To their surprise the dogs reacted more violently to the second than to the first shot and, in fact, died quite unexpectedly. It seemed that the first injection had sensitized rather than immunized them. The doctors called this unexpected reaction *anaphylaxis* to contrast with what they expected to occur, namely *prophylaxis*. It is a violent reaction such as this which occurs in the exceptional individual who is sensitive to a bee sting when he is stung for a second time or sensitive to penicillin when he is given a second shot.

Such an individual is usually not aware that he is allergic to the bee sting or to penicillin because he did not have a violent reaction after his first sting or shot, but within seconds or minutes of receiving his second or subsequent sting or shot, he may become flushed, and start to sweat, his chest and throat may become so tight that he cannot breathe, his blood pressure may fall, and he may die. If the patient is in the hospital being given penicillin, a timely injection of epinephrine will probably save him; if he is away from the hospital, he will either have recovered or have died by the time help is available.

If your child is allergic to bee, wasp, yellow jacket or hornet stings, arrange for him to be desensitized, and always carry epinephrine around with you when near bees or wasps. Epinephrine is available in *emergency kits*. Ask your doctor for a prescription for such a kit. Anaphylaxis is rare, but it is both frightening and dangerous. As for penicillin, make sure, if your child is allergic to penicillin, that anyone looking after him knows this, and as an extra precaution, give him a suitably worded bracelet to wear.

Contactants

Allergic individuals, in addition to reacting to things inhaled, ingested, and injected, occasionally react to things with which they are in contact, and these include everything from hair dyes and cosmetics to rings, zippers, and materials such as wool. A list would be meaningless for it would include almost everything under the sun. Sometimes these reactions seem to be allergic, as when a child develops a rash when he has been in contact with poison ivy or hives on his legs after walking through grass. Sometimes the reactions seem to be the result of irritation, but even in these cases the baby's skin must be unduly sensitive if it reacts so vigorously to a mild soap or bland oil; mothers often develop this kind of rash on their hands from contact with detergents. Whatever the mechanism, avoid the irritant or allergen; or if you do not know what it is, contact your doctor, and between the two of you, you should be able to sort out the problem.

Infections and Asthma

The onset of a cold is often the first indication that a child is going to have an attack of asthma, and as he usually seems very susceptible to colds, he will probably have frequent attacks of asthma. Colds, it is commonly believed, are due to infections. It is natural therefore to suppose that the child is allergic to infections. And though many people still believe this, there are one or two good reasons for questioning its validity.

When a germ enters the body to cause an illness, it usually does so once but rarely repeatedly. The normal child, for example, develops red measles once, but will rarely if ever develop red measles again let alone again and again. This is not because he will not be exposed to the measles virus again, because he will. In fact he will probably meet it whenever there is an epidemic, every two to three years, throughout his childhood.

The first time that he meets this germ he is unprepared, he is caught, as it were, with his pants down, and the virus is able to multiply in his tissues and to make him ill before his own defenses can be mobilized. However, the second time the virus enters his nose and lungs, his defenses are already alerted. He will not become ill; in fact, he will probably not know that his defenses have had a battle at all, but we will be pretty sure that they have because his younger brother has gone down with measles, and the two sleep in the same bedroom. If we had tested his blood before and after this contact, we would probably have found that his antibodies to the measles virus had suddenly increased, undeniable evidence of a silent victory. The same germ does not usually cause repeated illness in children with intact immunological systems. Once is enough, say the body's defenses.

A number of years ago, when it was thought that infections were commonly responsible for triggering off attacks of asthma, many children were given courses of bacterial vaccines. Some of the children improved, but so do many asthmatics who are not given vaccines. When groups of vaccinated and unvaccinated asthmatics were compared, it was found that there was no appreciable difference between them. The vaccine had either not helped, or the children had been given a vaccine against the wrong germs. We think the former explanation the more probable.

As this line of attack had failed, other children with this same type of so-called *infectious asthma* were given repeated injections of gamma globulin, hoping in this way to provide them with ammunition to hold their colds in check—but again with no obvious benefit. It is nevertheless possible that the exceptional child is allergic to *infectious agents*.

It was at about this time that we came across a family who seemed always to be catching colds; one child in particular had one cold after another, and with every cold he developed a cough. He was a frail little child. "He catches one cold after another from our baby-sitter," his mother would say. As he had had this problem ever since he was born, we felt we could hardly blame the baby-sitter.

We suspected that the child was allergic to something. Could he possibly be allergic to milk? There was only one way to find out and that was to take him off all milk and dairy products. This we did. The transformation was remarkable. He lost his susceptibility to colds, his appetite and color improved, and he put on weight. He has since developed one or two other allergies, but he still has to stay off milk if he wants to remain well. Some of his colds were no doubt due to germs, but most were a manifestation of his allergy.

Not long afterwards we saw another child, this time a girl who was almost a year old. She had been in and out of hospital nine times with pneumonia. Just before each attack, she would catch a cold; the cold would settle on her chest, her temperature would rise, and soon afterwards she would be in hospital in an oxygen tent. "But when she caught her last cold," her mother added, "I took her right off milk, and the cold never settled on her chest. I did not even have to call my doctor."

"Why did you take her off milk?" I asked.

"I know from my own experience," she replied, "that when I catch a cold, it will settle on my chest, unless I stop drinking milk. So I wondered whether milk might not be aggravating Brenda's chest and turning her colds into pneumonia."

"Well, why are you worried about her now?"

"Because she seems to be getting pneumonia again."

"Are you still giving her milk?" I could not help asking.

"Yes" came the answer.

"Why?"

"Well, when she had recovered, I thought I should put her back on the bottle. Milk is supposed to be good for you." That was Brenda's mother's big mistake. If you want to keep an allergic baby or child well, keep him away from everything that he is allergic to. This is the golden rule of allergy.

I could relate many more similar histories. Some mothers find it almost unbelievable and so did I, once. But do not assume that milk is always to blame. Any food to which a child is allergic can cause runny noses and bronchitis, and so can house dust, feathers, dog dander, and a host of other things. If your child has frequent colds and bronchitis, he is almost certainly allergic, possibly to foods, possibly to inhalants, possibly to germs, possibly to all three.

Sad to say the picture is not always as simple as the stories I have told you would suggest. Recently a group of Australian doctors have rechecked children who had been admitted to hospital early in life, before they were two years old, with bronchiolitis due to a virus. Half of this group of children subsequently had spells of wheezing or asthma; this is many more than would have been expected by chance. So it would seem that children with respiratory allergies are unduly susceptible to infectious bronchiolitis. Not all bronchiolitis is allergy, but repeated attacks of bronchiolitis usually indicate that the child has a basic underlying allergy.

Physical Factors and Allergy

There are several other factors which, by themselves, may cause allergic reactions. These are cold, heat, sunshine, and exercise. Cold and exercise more commonly aggravate asthma, and cold more commonly aggravates eczema. The child who remains symptom free in a warm house may begin to wheeze when he goes outside into the cold frosty air, or when he starts to run around with his playmates. But in addition to this, contact with cold water or cold air may bring on hives. If such a person exposes his whole body to the cold, for example by plunging into the cold sea for a swim, his whole body may become swollen with giant hives, and he may collapse. One child we have seen would have an attack of asthma if she drank a glass of cold water. Exposure to sunshine, quite apart from sunburn, may also cause urticaria, but usually only where the skin is exposed. Similarly exercise alone, in certain rare individuals who are otherwise free from asthma, may induce an attack of asthma.

Psychological Factors and Asthma

An attack of asthma can be, and often is, a terrifying experience; for, during an attack, the control of a vital function, *breathing out and breathing in,* seems to be taken over by an unseen enemy. The asthmatic has literally to fight for his breath, to fight for the right to breathe. It is not surprising, therefore, that any child who has had an attack of asthma is disturbed and may become a psychological problem. This applies particularly to the child who has had repeated attacks of asthma, especially if they have necessitated frequent admissions to hospital.

Many, if not most, parents of asthmatic children also become concerned and may even become overly anxious. And no wonder, for the attacks seem to descend on the child out of the blue. When neither the doctor nor the parents have an adequate explanation for these attacks, psychological causes are often invoked. We doctors are very much aware of the importance of psychological factors but feel that we should not incriminate them until we have excluded all other possibilities; for a psychological explanation, if wrong, is fair neither to the child nor to the parents.

One reason often put forward for implicating the parents is that the child often seems to get better remarkably quickly when he is taken away from home. In the hospital his wheezing quickly subsides, helped by modern treatment. When he is discharged, he may, to all intents and appearances, be normal, but before long the wheezing returns and so do his visits to the doctor's office or the hospital emergency room. Another reason for implicating the parents is that severely affected children when sent away to special homes for asthmatics often make remarkable recoveries. They may even be able to stop taking their medicines. Both these observations suggest that contact with the parents, possibly because they are so anxious, induces further attacks of asthma. This reasoning is not always fair to the parent or child for the house may be full of a hundred and one other things, from dust to pets and molds, that can also induce asthma.

An acquaintance of mine used to have severe attacks of asthma as a child. These attacks were frequent and severe until he went away to boarding school. His attacks immediately stopped. It was assumed that this was because his school was in a healthy location by the sea. His next attack of asthma, and I think his last, occurred years later when, as a medical student, he was dissecting a rabbit. As a little boy he had had pet rabbits. When he was sent away to school, his rabbits were returned to their maker. When he himself returned home for his holidays, he remained free from asthma. It was contact with rabbits which had brought on the attacks of asthma.

We recently saw a child who had had repeated attacks of asthma since early infancy. Her parents, who taught in a school in a relatively inaccessible part of the Canadian North, decided to leave their daughter with grandparents while her problem was being sorted out. We suspected that milk might be to blame, for her symptoms had dated from infancy, so we put her on a diet free from milk and dairy products. She became symptom free. We placed her back on milk, but the asthma did not return. One day the TV repairman called to repair the television set. As he started to work, he lit a cigarette; within a few minutes Darlene began to wheeze. This child's asthma had subsided for the first time when she was separated from her concerned and naturally anxious parents, not because their anxiety was making her ill, but because she was allergic to smoke from their cigarettes.

We have had another little patient who only developed asthma when in contact with her grandmother. This little child remained perfectly well in her own home, but every time she went with her mother to visit her grandmother in a distant city, she had an attack of asthma and ended up in the emergency department receiving epinephrine. It was thought that the child could not tolerate her own mother transferring her affection from her daughter to her daughter's granny. Tests showed that Darlene was allergic to horse hair. In point of fact her wheezing would start when she sat in a chair stuffed with horse hair in the basement of her grandmother's home.

If it is easy to provide psychological explanations for asthma due to exposure to rabbit fur and horse dander, how much easier must it be to provide similar explanations for a common problem like enuresis which usually has no very obvious explanation anyway? The example which I gave earlier of the child's enuresis apparently being precipitated by her return to school is a case in point. Although I have emphasized that it is easy to substitute psychological for valid explanations, this is not to deny that psychological factors are important. They are important, but they tend more often to compound rather than cause the problem.

Chapter V

IMMUNOLOGY AND ALLERGY

Allergy and immunology are closely related. It is for this reason that if you are to understand your allergies, you must also learn a little immunology.

Immunology began as the study of the body's defenses against the germs which try to invade and overcome it. It was then extended to include, because the reactions are essentially the same, the study of the body's reactions to all foreign substances, not only to germs such as diphtheria and to the diphtheria toxin itself, but also to things like egg protein, horse serum, animal dander, and to foods such as crab and strawberry for these sometimes cause hives.

Reactions to horse serum came to the fore because many people used to be given horse serum containing diphtheria or tetanus antitoxin, and though the antitoxin helped people to recover, some reacted violently because they had apparently developed a hypersensitivity to the horse serum. The study of immunology has recently been extended to include the study of the body's defenses against its own cells when they become cancerous or malignant. Allergy developed as the study of those unusual reactions which occur when the body becomes sensitive rather than immune to whatever it is exposed. Our immunological knowledge is still far from complete, but I will try to paint in the broad outlines.

The evolutionary process, as you are only too well aware, is the result of a struggle for existence, the fittest only surviving. When Darwin first put forward this hypothesis, he was thinking mainly, if not entirely, in terms of the animals and plants which he had studied. He had noticed that some animals survived because they had developed special coloring and merged into the background, remaining unnoticed by their enemies; other animals survived because their great speeds enabled them to escape from their enemies; the giraffe survived because he was able to reach leaves inaccessible to other leaf-eating animals; the desert cactus survived because its thick-skinned foliage conserved the water extracted from the arid soil. To survive and reproduce it was essential that the whole individual, animal or plant, should develop special skills such as speed, strong teeth, protective coloring or protective covering, quills for the porcupine and hide for the rhinocerous, or special weapons such as venom to enable him to compete for survival with his neighbors.

But this visible struggle for survival was not the only struggle taking place within and among the various species. It was accompanied by an equally important but less obvious struggle between individuals and unseen enemies such as viruses, bacteria, and worms. Big teeth and powerful claws were not only powerless, they were useless against such enemies. New highly sophisticated tools were required for these enemies. Immunology began as the study of this interaction between the more highly developed animal species and the simpler organisms which were trying to live in their tissues where there was an unlimited supply of nourishment.

Animals and plants also have a third enemy with whom they must deal; this is the most difficult of all enemies to handle; it is the traitor from within. As you are aware, new cells are constantly being formed in the body to replace old cells which have run their course. These new cells must be exact replicas of their parent cells if they are to carry out their duties efficiently or if the body is to remain healthy and strong. Fortunately they nearly always are, but every now and then, a new cell is born which is deformed, just as occasionally a new baby is born which is deformed; such a cell is usually ill-fitted to survive, and if so, it dies.

Sometimes, however, it is strong and aggressive, but having a different constitution from its parent cell, it pays no attention to the needs of the body as a whole; it no longer does what is expected of it. Instead it grows and multiplies to its heart's content; in a word, it becomes *malignant*. For individuals to survive any length of time, it is essential that such cells should be detected and killed as soon as they appear. How does the body handle these unseen enemies, those from without, the bacteria, viruses, and worms, and those from within, the traitorous cancer cells?

In the bone marrow, where cells that are found in the blood are made, originate the cells, called lymphocytes, which play a key role in the body's defenses. One of their most important duties is to learn to recognize and distinguish friend from foe; for only when they have done this, can they turn their attention to the enemy and annihilate him. They have therefore first to be taught the salient features of the cells in their own body so that they can distinguish them from their enemies.

The special lymphocytes, we will call them the *soldier cells*, whose duty it is to fight the enemy from without—the bacteria and viruses—are sent for their training to their own Military Academy, the equivalent of Aldershot in England and West Point in the United States and The Royal Military College in Canada. Where in the body is this academy? We are not yet certain, but it is probably either in the bone marrow or in the lining of the bowel. In birds we know it is in a special organ in the bowel called the Bursa of Fabricius. Wherever it is in man, the cells are here grouped into combat forces, some become shock troops to withstand the first onslought, others become front line troops to blunt the initial attack, while the majority form the reserves used to overpower the enemy.

They are also provided with the necessary weapons best suited to destroy the bacteria and viruses they expect to encounter. The various ammunitions which these soldiers, and the workers (plasma cells), make in the factories are the missiles and bullets with which the enemy is made powerless if not destroyed. These are called Immunoglobulins. The shock troops, the cells called up in an emergency when the enemy is seen for the first time, make Immunoglobulin M. They hold the enemy in check while the reserves are brought up, and the army as a whole is mobilized. The ammunition of the reserves is called Immunoglobulin G.

Calling up the reserves and preparing the ammunition usually takes ten to fourteen days; this takes place during the incubation period of an illness. When the reserves join the field of battle and while the battle is being fought, the patient usually feels ill. Once it is over, he quickly recovers. Babies, before they are delivered, are provided by the mother with a generous supply of the ammunition, Immunoglobulin G, so that they have a ready source of this and are able to repel most of the invaders that may try to attack them at this time.

There is another class of soldier who dwells in the lining of the nose and bronchial tubes, and of the stomach and bowel, and bladder. This soldier makes a special kind of ammunition called secretory Immunoglobulin A. This immunoglobulin is processed as it passes through the cells into the bronchial tubes, bowel and bladder; it is made resistant to the action of digestive juices and germs. It lies in wait, like the booby traps and antitank mines laid by soldiers in the field, for the unwary germ trying to enter the body. It forms the first line of the body's defense, repelling the potential invader before he has a chance to penetrate the tissues of his intended victim.

Two more kinds of ammunition are made by the soldier cells, the lymphocytes, and both are present in relatively small amounts. They are called Immunoglobulin D and Immunoglobulin E. We do not, at the present time, know whether Immunoglobulin D has any special function, but at least it probably adds a little variety to the defenses of the host, like the big guns which back up the mortar fire. Immunoglobulin E seems to have as its special function the defeat and destruction of the many varieties of worms, roundworms, hookworms, tapeworms, and so on that try to make their home in the human host.

The cells whose task it is to protect the body from the enemy within, cancer, have a very different task to perform. They go for their training to their own special academy, the *thymus*. In Canada we would call these cells the Mounties, and we would send them to Regina for their training. In the States they would be members of the Federal Bureau of Investigation. In England they would form the backbone of Scotland Yard. Here the cells are taught the salient features of the cells they expect to meet in their own body so that they can quickly identify and distinguish them from any antisocial cancer cells that they may encounter. By the same token they are quickly able to identify any foreign cells which a hopeful surgeon may wish to graft onto or introduce into their own body. They also play an important role in the fight against some virus infections and tuberculosis.

The reader is aware that each individual has his own blood group, just as he has his own name; each individual likewise has his own *cell group*, and just as no two people, apart from identical twins, have exactly the same blood groups, so probably no two people, again identical twins excepted, have exactly the same cell groups. The police cells are able to spot and, with the help of ancillary forces, kill off any cancer cells that may develop in their respective bodies.

Sometimes, particularly in old age, the police cells are caught napping and do not discover the multiplying cancer cells until it is too late, until the cancer is so widespread that it cannot be defeated. A long, drawnout battle may ensue, but without the intervention of x-rays, surgery, or special drugs, the cancer cells usually win. In little children the first cancer cells probably originate long before the baby is born, and at this time the police cells do not realize that they are in fact malignant; they believe them to be harmless, and for this reason make no attempt to destroy them. It may be for this reason that cancer tends to run such a rapid course in little children.

In order to do their utmost to ensure victory, both the police and soldiers need additional support; their immunoglobulin ammunition alone is not enough, so they also indulge in chemical warfare. The chemicals they make help in the following ways. One chemical attracts cells called macrophages to where the action is. These cells can engulf, digest, and destroy germs. A second chemical keeps the macrophages and polymorphs, an important group of white cells in the blood, on the field of battle so that there is no danger of it being lost through desertions or shortage of troops. A third stops the multiplication of viruses, keeping down the number of the enemy and preventing them bringing up reinforcements. A fourth is a powerful poison killing germs outright, a fifth stimulates colleagues to make more ammunition, and a sixth makes the walls of the blood vessels more permeable so that the soldiers can get through to the tissue spaces where the germs are holding out.

These chemicals are made by many of the soldiers, but some of the troops have an additional cannister of powerful chemicals called complement. One of these chemicals attracts the macrophages and polymorphonuclear leukocytes to the scene of battle where they are needed; the remainder contribute in new ways to the destruction of the enemy. A second chemical latches onto bacteria and viruses and straps them to cells such as platelets and red cells, probably to prevent them escaping from the scene of battle; they can then be destroyed locally and cannot spread to other parts of the body.

A third chemical has a powerful action on the protective covering of bacteria; the body has difficulty in destroying some bacteria because they have such tough *armour plating,* the plating is eroded by this chemical, and when the protective shield has been penetrated, other white cells, called macrophages and polymorphs, can ingest them. A fourth chemical liberates a powerful substance called histamine from special little containers in mast cells and basophils where it is stored; we will desribe the actions of this chemical a little later.

A fifth, and very important chemical, is actually able to pierce the walls of bacteria and foreign cells, literally disembowelling them; their contents leak out onto the field of battle. Our soldiers and police are, luckily for us, not only extraordinarily thorough, but also quite merciless. The destruction of bacteria and viruses is not quite as simple as at one time it appeared, but it is carried out with remarkable efficiency.

When the battle is over and the victory has been won, the soldiers put away their weapons, but not before a record has been made by intelligence officers, called memory cells, of the most effective ammunition to use against this enemy. The immunoglobulin ammunition, which the body manufactures, is prepared especially for each and every enemy encountered. The bullets that effectively kill, for example, the red measles virus, although similar in some respects to those that kill the German measles virus, differ in certain essentials, so much so in fact that they would not even give the German measles virus a headache.

It is vital, therefore, if the body is to be spared a major battle with the red measles virus every time it meets it, and this is every two or three years, that it should remember exactly which bullet to manufacture for each and every germ it encounters. And this is where the memory cells, the intelligence officers, come in.

Whenever the germ is encountered a second, third, or fourth time, the soldiers which have made a specialty of fighting the red measles virus are immediately called on to produce their special ammunition. They are helped in this task by the workers, the plasma cells, in the factories. This reaction is so swift that the virus does not have a chance to multiply. The body is spared a second battle and its accompanying illness. In order to make doubly certain of victory, some of the soldiers are constantly circulating round the body with their ammunition at the ready, like warplanes on constant vigil, so that they can put an end to any stray red measles virus that may come their way.

Modern immunization procedures have protected most children in many parts of the world from the more common infectious diseases, so much so that big epidemics of poliomyelitis, whooping cough, diphtheria, and red and German measles should never occur again, at least not on the scale that they did in the past. Protection against these diseases now follows either a series of *shots* given at the clinic or doctor's office, or doses of the organisms, as in the case of poliomyelitis ,which are swallowed. Diphtheria is dangerous mainly because the germ produces a powerful toxin or poison which may damage the heart and nervous system; tetanus is likewise dangerous because it too produces a toxin; the tetanus toxin makes nerves unduly sensitive, resulting in convulsions and *lock-jaw*.

Protection is ensured by injecting the toxins, first made harmless by previous modifications with chemicals, of diphtheria and tetanus. In their harmless form the toxins are called toxoids. The soldier cells naturally become aware of the toxoids and promptly start to make the necessary ammunition, Immunoglobulins A and G for the most part, to neutralize them. Booster injections of toxoid should be given from time to time to keep the soldiers and intelligence officers on the alert. Protection against poliomyelitis and red measles was first ensured by injections of dead virus, but the response on the part of the soldiers was not always sufficiently brisk to ensure that there would always be plenty available to tackle the live poliomyelitis and red measles viruses when they came along. Attempts were therefore made to modify the viruses, making them harmless but not killing them.

Injections of these viruses, especially in the case of red measles, may cause minor reactions, comparable to a very minor attack of measles, but the soldiers react more vigorously and build up a bigger supply of ammunition. The intelligence officers also take greater notice, and when the real viruses are encountered at a later date, the body reacts as quickly as it would have done had it already had a real infection, and no one even suspects that it has fought off the measles or polio viruses.

In this brief review I have indicated that the police and soldiers have different fields of action, and though this is to a great extent true, it should be added that they do not work completely independently of each other. Their work often brings them together, and when this happens, they naturally cooperate and help each other.

We mentioned earlier that ammunition is made by the soldiers not only against germs, but also against any foreign dead matter that may get into the body. Most individuals make the common types of ammunition, Immunoglobulin G, A, and M to these substances, but they may also make tiny amounts of Immunoglobulin E. Most of this Immunoglobulin E is carried round in the circulation ready to render harmless any of the foreign proteins and other substances that may enter the body, but some becomes attached, why we do not know, to a special groups of cells called mast cells . . . and basophils.

These cells resemble, in many respects, the polymorphs, but unlike the polymorphs, they contain a powerful chemical called histamine. When the Immunoglobulin E on their surface comes in contact with the foreign material that caused their initial development, the mast cell immediately discharges the very powerful histamine, mentioned earlier, into the surrounding tissue spaces. Histamine in small amounts helps in the battle against germs by making blood vessels dilate so that the white cells and chemicals can quickly reach the scene of the conflict and then make their way through the vessel walls into the tissue spaces.

But histamine also acts on other tissues. It makes the bronchial tubes contract, causing wheezing, blood vessels called capillaries to dilate causing hives, and the blood vessels in the head to dilate causing a headache, the stomach or bowel to contract causing vomiting or diarrhea. It is for this reason that the allergic individual has such unpleasant reactions whenever he meets whatever he is allergic to. When I eat an egg, I not only enjoy it, but I am left with a happy, well-satisfied feeling, but I have a colleague who avoids eating even traces of egg; for if he eats no more than the tiny amount of egg that is found in a cookie his lips and tongue begin to tingle, his nose then runs, his eyes water, his chest tightens, and he begins to wheeze. His stomach is also upset, and he begins to vomit.

These reactions occur whenever even infinitesimally small particles of egg get into his circulation. The particles of egg are carried swiftly around his body and his defenses, having encountered egg on a previous occasion, are already primed for action. The mast cells, carrying their anti-egg ammunition in the form of Immunoglobulin E, latch onto the egg and then immediately discharge the chemical histamine into the circulation. It is the histamine that causes the unpleasant reactions that make him ill.

Sometimes the liberation of histamine into the circulation is so swift, generalized, and massive that it leads to death. This violent reaction is called anaphylaxis. This type of reaction may occur in those who are allergic to penicillin when given a shot of penicillin and in those stung by bees who are allergic to bee stings. More commonly, however, the reaction is localized, as though only the mast cells in special places were prepared to joust with the *invader*. When this is so, the person develops only local symptoms. His eyes and nose may run, and his nose may become stuffed up; he develops hay fever. His lungs may fill up with mucous and his bronchial tubes tighten; he develops asthma. His skin may develop welts and itch; he develops hives. For similar reasons the vessels in his head may dilate, and he will develop a throbbing headache —migraine.

We still have much to learn about the allergic reaction. Histamine is not the only powerful chemical to be liberated in this reaction, but it is the one we know most about. Immunoglobulin E and mast cells are probably not the only ammunition and not the only cells to be involved, but again they are the ones that at present we know most about.

Chapter VI

IMMUNOGLOBULIN E

I mentioned in the last chapter that the survival of any one species depended on its ability to compete successfully for the necessities of life, and that in this competition we, in common with many other animals, had to fight three battles; the first against other animals, the second against viruses, bacteria, and parasites such as malaria and worms, and the third against cancer. The first battle against other animals we have, by our ingenuity, won so successfully that we have actually exterminated some of the less vigorous adversaries such as the auk and the passenger pigeon. We have enslaved others, the slavery sometimes being quite benevolent as with the horse, and sometimes purely mercenary, as with the cow and hen. The animals that are neither extinct nor enslaved are sometimes allowed to roam free or are sometimes placed in cages for our gratification.

The war against viruses, bacteria, and parasites is being won, for we have learned how to forewarn our defenses for the battles that lie ahead by procedures called *immunization*. We have also acquired powerful new tools in the form of antibiotics to supplement our own defenses. The third battle, against cancer, is still in its infancy. In parenthesis I should add that survival in the world of nature is best assured not by confrontation but by accommodation. Plants and animals do not fight each other, they support each other; one provides shade, shelter, and nourishment while the other returns the nourishment in valuable droppings. In another context many germs which live in your bowel and mine pay for their accommodation by providing us with free vitamins, while we provide them with a relatively sheltered and nutritious environment. Our chief fear for the human race is that the weapons which it has engineered for its own survival will be utilized for its own destruction. Man is in danger of having everything except common sense.

In this struggle for survival it sometimes happens that a useful acquisition may, with a change of environment, become either unnecessary or even a handicap. The penguin, for example, at one stage of his development could fly, but in the icy Antarctic wings became unnecessary and in fact became a handicap. There were few predators from whom to fly, no trees on which to perch, no midges to catch, and there were even no places to fly to. So the penguins adapted to the world of snow and ice and ocean and survived. Webbed feet and flippers replaced talons and wings. To bring the simile nearer home, we can see the need for analogous changes in our own development.

The malarial parasite, as you are aware, spends part of his life cycle in the human red blood cell. Some Negroes, by chance, developed a new form of hemoglobin; we call it hemoglobin *S;* the *S* is for sickle because red cells which contain this type of hemoglobin lose their round shapes and look like sickles. This type of hemoglobin does not provide the malignant tertian malarial parasite with a suitable home, and so such parasites when they enter the blood stream containing cells which are full of sickle hemoglobin are not as likely to survive. The host is more likely to recover from his infection. Unfortunately sickle hemoglobin is not the best of hemoglobins with which to pack red cells, for as we have already indicated, it tends to distort them so that they do not circulate as readily; they tend to clog up smaller blood vessels.

Nevertheless, Negroes living in highly malarious areas are better off if some of their red cells contain sickle hemoglobin than they are if all their red cells contain only the normal, so-called hemoglobin A. They are also better off than those whose cells contain only sickle hemoglobin; these people develop sickle cell disease and have a diminished chance of survival. In a malarial area, other things being equal, the race's chance of survival is increased if some, at least, of the population packs sickle hemoglobin into some of its red cells. But should malaria be exterminated or should the Negro move into a nonmalarial area, as he did when he moved to the United States, sickle hemoglobin loses all its advantages and literally becomes a millstone around the Negro's neck.

The ammunition which we have called Immunoglobulin E may, in this respect, resemble sickle hemoglobin. IgE, as it is called for short, is present in the blood in greatest amounts in people who have either allergies or worms. Worms are not an important cause of disease or illness in countries with good hygiene, but they are elsewhere, particularly in the tropics. Some worms, such as the thread or pin worm, seem to live harmlessly in the bowel and probably do little more than cause an irritation around the anus when they come out at night to lay their eggs. But the irritation is enough to make the child reach down and scratch himself, and later, unwittingly transfer the eggs to his mouth so that they can make their way down to the bowel and develop into new thread worms.

Other worms, however, are not so harmless; they actually invade the body's tissues. The round worm, which may look like an ordinary earthworm, lives, like the thread worm, in the bowel, but its larvae penetrate the bowel wall and enter the blood stream; they make their way to the lungs where they mature and sometimes cause pneumonia. They then climb up the wind pipe and down the esophagus to find a haven once again in the bowel.

A third group of worms lives entirely in the tissues as larvae, eggs, and adults. Some develop big cysts, called hydatid cysts, which may cause disease in the lungs, liver, and elsewhere. Other types of worms cause little cysts in the muscles and even in the brain. British soldiers in the past used often to acquire this kind of infection in India; many were invalided home with epilepsy. Other worms cause severe disease in the bladder, spleen, liver, and bowel. One disease they cause is schistosomiasis. There are 200 million people in the world today with this kind of disease.

It is quite obvious that in many parts of the world worms once posed or still pose a real threat to mankind. It is thought that Immunoglobulin E is the most effective ammunition that we have to ward off second attacks by this kind of enemy. In fact Immunoglobulin E may well have been developed as a special weapon to prevent worms or their larvae from wriggling through the bowel wall or skin. The histamine liberated in the bowel would, among other things, cause diarrhea. This would help to dispose of the worms by hurrying them through to the outside world.

Unfortunately Immunoglobulin E is sometimes directed not only at dangerous worms, but also, in the allergic individual, at beneficial foods, and otherwise harmless dusts and pollens. When this is the case, Immunoglobulin E in the bowel tries to get rid of the food. The innocent host finds that the egg which he should enjoy makes him vomit or gives him diarrhea. Similarly when Immunoglobulin E meets substances against which it has made ammunition in the skin, a minor explosion, eczema or urticaria, results. The same train of events occurs in the lungs, resulting in asthma.

It would seem that Immunoglobulin E, like sickle hemoglobin, may be a mixed blessing. Those among us who are best equipped to fight the lowly worm, which may no longer threaten us, are probably those most likely to be handicapped by allergies.

Chapter VII

ARE ALLERGIES INHERITED?

As you are aware, many of our characteristics are genetically determined, and for this reason are passed on from one generation to the next. Some characteristics, or traits as they are often called, are controlled by a single gene. A simple example of such a trait is the ability to taste a bitter chemical compound called phenylthiourea. This ability was discovered accidentally when a scientist who had synthesized it was surprised to find that a colleague said it tasted bitter, while he himself found it tasteless. Most Europeans, about 70 percent, can detect even traces of it, 30 percent cannot.

The ability to taste phenylthiourea is transmitted as a dominant trait. If one child in a family can detect it, then one or other parent must also be able to detect it; if neither parent can taste it, none of their children will be able to taste it. The transmission of other characteristics, for example that of height, is not determined by a single gene, for if it were, we would all, like Gregor Mendel's peas, be tall, short, or halfway in between. Heights are determined by many genes. The effects of these genes are modified by such factors as nutrition and illness because both influence normal growth and development, and by sex, girls are usually shorter than boys, as well as by the normal working of the endocrine glands and other organs.

To what extent are allergies transmitted? Allergies are very common. In almost every family group, if grandparents, parents, and children are included, someone will be found with an allergy, if not with an allergic problem. Nevertheless, allergy problems seem to be concentrated in certain families. Some families are plagued with them, others are relatively free. We have recently studied a series of over 700 children, some of whom had allergies and some had not. We found that the children with allergies were more likely to have parents and brothers and sisters with allergies than were the children who were free from allergies. This suggests that there are genetic factors which predispose towards the development of allergies.

In keeping with these observations is the finding that the amounts of Immunoglobulin E in the blood seem to be under genetic control. This has been shown very clearly by studies on identical twins by Dr. Hamburger and his colleagues. We know that levels of Immunoglobulin E are clearly related to allergy, those with high levels of Immunoglobulin E being much more likely to develop allergies than those with low levels. We suspect therefore that not only allergies, but also Immunoglobulin E levels run in families.

Studies with identical twins have also shown that it is not just the tendency to develop allergies in general that is transmitted, but that it is also the tendency to develop a specific allergy, asthma, or hay fever, for example. If one of identical twins develops asthma, or hay fever, or eczema, his identical twin is two to three times as likely to develop the same problem as is the twin who is not identical.

We can say therefore that not only does the tendency to develop an allergy run in families, but so does the tendency to develop a specific allergy. Asthma may run in one family, hay fever in another, eczema in a third, and migraine in a fourth, though in each group of families there will also be relatives with other kinds of allergies. Allergies, however, are not transmitted in a simple way, like the ability to taste phenylthiourea, but as yet we do not know what factors control their transmission.

The only allergic problem that we have studied in detail, from this point of view, has been that related to bed-wetting. Bed-wetting is often due to a bladder allergy. Bed-wetting too tends to run in families. The mothers and fathers of bed-wetters are five times as likely to have wet the bed when they were young as are the parents of children who do not wet the bed. Brothers and sisters of bed-wetters are also more likely to wet the bed than are the brothers and sisters of children who are dry at night. But the inheritance of an allergy is not as simple as that of being able or unable to taste phenylthiourea, for if one of identical twins can taste it, the other will always also be able to taste it.

Whether a person develops an allergy depends not only on his genetic makeup, but also on whether he is exposed to the allergen to which he has made or is making his Immunoglobulin E ammunition. For example, a child born in New Hampshire, whose parents are incapacitated by hay fever in late summer when the ragweed season bursts on them, might also develop ragweed hay fever were he to remain in New Hampshire. But if when he is two years old, his parents were to move to California where ragweed is not a problem, he himself would not be exposed to ragweed and might never develop hay fever. It may never be known whether he inherited the capability of developing ragweed hay fever. By the same token a new arrival in the prairie provinces may develop asthma for the first time from grain dust. On close questioning, he may state that he is the only asthmatic in his family. This may be true, but we cannot be sure that his parents and brothers and sisters would have remained free from asthma had they too moved to the prairies.

A third factor that makes the unravelling of genetic factors difficult is that allergies have a habit of suddenly appearing and just as suddenly of disappearing. Eczema is commonest in infancy. A child as a baby may develop eczema when given egg, this is quite common in our experience, but when she is older, she may be able to take an egg without developing a rash; she has *grown out of* her egg allergy. Later she marries, and has a baby of her own; her baby too develops eczema when given egg, but she herself is unaware that she once was allergic to eggs. She will not be able to provide the geneticist with the information he is looking for.

We should next ask ourselves whether those with allergies can develop allergies to any and everything, or whether they are capable of developing allergies to only a limited number of things.

A definite answer cannot be given to this question but the following observations may provide clues. Most individuals with allergies are keenly aware that they have more than one allergy, that they are allergic to several things. One person may be allergic to milk, tomato, and corn, another to pollen grains and house dust, but even though most allergic individuals are allergic to more than one thing, none are allergic to everything.

I, for one, have certainly not yet met anyone who was allergic to everything in his environment. It is felt by some, however, that the allergic individual will develop allergic reactions to any and everything if he is exposed to it in sufficient quantities and for a sufficiently long time. They say that the individual who moves to California, where there is little if any ragweed, to escape his annual ragweed hay fever, inevitably becomes a victim of Bermuda grass, which is prevalent there. This has been the experience of some individuals but certainly not of all.

When we look into this problem in greater detail, we cannot fail to realize that most patients are remarkably selective in the choice of their allergies. They are by no means most sensitive to the *thing* or *things* to which they are most exposed. The child may be able to play freely with the dog or cat in his home and yet wheeze as soon as he puts his head in the barn. The same is applicable to foods. Not every child who is allergic to cow's milk becomes allergic to soya when given it in equally generous amounts; in fact, only about one child in five does so. I have come across one or two children who appeared to be allergic to almost every food they were offered, but always one food was found which could be tolerated, and this food could be eaten day after day without causing an untoward reaction.

One child who was sensitive to all formulas, to soya, to most meats, and most cereals, was able to tolerate wheat, and because his diet was very limited, he lived on wheat. He has not shown any signs of becoming sensitive to it. He has also shown no sign of being allergic to inhalants. There are still many things which do not upset him. It would seem that each individual is born with a limited number of potential allergies, but whether he will or will not develop these depends both on whether he is exposed to them, and also on how often and to what degree he is exposed to them.

A second great variable in allergic individuals is the degree of their sensitivity. Some people are upset by traces of a food, some only by comparatively large amounts. It is a commonly held belief, and a mistaken one, that the allergic person is always so responsive to the allergen that even traces will upset him. This is not true. Some people are much more sensitive than others. A onetime neighbor, the mother of five boys who were all allergic to milk, vomited so forcefully when she herself was first offered cow's milk as a baby that she was obviously very sensitive to milk.

One of her sons when first offered cow's milk refused to drink it, but when a little was forced between his lips, he too, vomited copiously. Both mother and son were so sensitive to cow's milk that traces of it made them ill. By contrast other children can take milk in moderate amounts and remain symptom free, but they, as we have seen, have to avoid milk as soon as they "catch a cold" or the cold will "settle on their chests." So it would seem that individuals are selective in the inhalants and foods to which they are sensitive, and they are also selective in the vigor with which they will respond to them.

Whether specific sensitivities are transmitted is still debatable. I have been interested in this subject for some time and have made a point of trying to find out if more than one member of the family was allergic to the same food. The food that I have studied most is cow's milk for the simple reason that it is the food which all adults either avoid or drink. It is, however, an unfortunate food to choose for it contains hundreds of different substances, to anyone of which allergies could develop.

In the example given above, two quite different substances in the milk might have caused the vomiting in the mother and her baby. Bearing these limitations in mind, we have come across many families in which more than one child was allergic to milk, and others in which a sensitivity to milk was present in two, three, or even four generations. This familial sensitivity is so common that, having detected it in a baby, one can usually unearth it in other members of the family.

The results of taking other members of the family off milk are sometimes surprising. I have learned much about the symptoms that foods can produce from this. One patient, a girl, was troubled by repeated spells of tummy pains. Such spells of pain are common in children and are regarded by some as being of no consequence. This child's spells of pain were so severe that her parents insisted on trying to determine the cause. After a very extensive negative *work-up,* in which even the lining of the bowel was examined, I decided to take her off milk and wheat. Her father was a great milk drinker who had frequent colds and sinus infections. Cow's milk is a common cause of this problem, so I also took him off milk.

The girl's spells of abdominal pain gradually subsided. They did not return when she was given wheat, but they did return when she was given even traces of milk. Bread made without milk, for example, caused no discomfort, but bread made with milk caused severe pain. I was not surprised when the father returned with a nose which no longer ran and with sinuses that were clear, and neither was he for that matter. But he was surprised to find that coming off milk caused a change in his bowel habits. He had always gone to the toilet two to three times day, he considered this natural, but when he stopped taking milk, he found that he had to go only once a day; his stools became formed.

Another change that he noticed was this, that previously he had been plagued by an *itchy bottom;* he was constantly having to hide behind doors to scratch himself, but now his bottom no longer itched. The bowels of both father and daughter were sensitive to milk; the milk caused a mild diarrhea in one and spells of abdominal pain, probably due to spasm, in the other. The father's nose was also sensitive to milk, the daughter's was not.

A better substance to study in an attempt to discover whether specific allergies are inherited is penicillin; for not only have many people had it and therefore know whether or not they are sensitive to it, but, unlike milk, it is a relatively simple substance. One cannot, unfortunately, go around giving penicillin to patients indiscriminately, particularly in allergic families, for some people who react to penicillin do so so violently that they are in danger of going into shock. People die of penicillin allergy every year. Nevertheless I have been impressed by the frequency with which penicillin sensitivities seem to run in families. I have encountered one family in which penicillin allergies were present in four generations.

From the practical point of view specific allergies run in families so frequently that the information they provide helps in the detection and management of allergic problems. Had Mrs. Q., the mother who vomited and whose baby vomited so copiously when given milk, realized that milk allergies ran in families, she herself would have been spared endless anxiety, and her children would have been spared innumerable illnesses and visits to doctors.

Two other problems complicate the study of the genetics of allergy. The first is that an individual person's allergies often come and go. Many patients with classical hay fever, for example, whose noses and eyes begin to run when exposed to pollen, may have their first allergic symptoms when they reach their teens. Their hay fever may persist indefinitely, but it may also go as suddenly and unexpectedly as it came. Women similarly may develop migraine at puberty and lose it at the menopause, or develop it for the first time at the menopause.

Finally we should mention that the same substance, a food or inhalant, may upset different parts of the body in different members of the family. When this happens, a familial sensitivity to a food may be present and remain unrecognized. One mother brought her 18-month-old child to me because she had a distended abdomen and was vomiting repeatedly. Her symptoms diminished when we took her off milk, but she continued to vomit from time to time at night, but only when given oats at suppertime. When she stopped taking oats, the vomiting subsided, as did the abdominal distention.

This child had a six-month-old baby sister who was having one cold after another; with each cold her ears would become inflamed. When her mother stopped giving milk to her, her *colds* also stopped, as did the inflammation of her ears. Oddly enough, or more correctly, as might be expected, this child's mother had a chronic allergic rhinitis. This rhinitis appeared to be aggravated by pregnancy; for when she was pregnant, she would develop repeated attacks of otitis media and would have to have her ear drums pierced and drained. She had the same problem as her baby daughter. She was not a great milk drinker, but she drank some milk each day, and when she was pregnant, she doubled up on her milk intake. When she too stopped drinking milk, her nose cleared, though not completely, for she also had other allergies, and her ears no longer became inflamed. Milk caused vomiting in one child and an allergic rhinitis in her sister and mother.

Another mother brought a six-month-old child to me with vomiting; again the vomiting was found to be due to cow's milk. This child had a sister who had intractable enuresis. I had seen her previously, but at that time I had not realized that enuresis might be an allergic problem. I thought it was a so-called developmental disorder which the child would outgrow. I had reassured her mother accordingly.

Later, when I discovered that she had a brother who was allergic to milk, and knowing that milk allergies often run in families, I wondered whether she too might not be sensitive to milk. Very reluctantly, not wanting to be thought too unconventional, I asked Mrs. L to take her enuretic daughter off milk and dairy products. This she did without saying a word to either the patient or to her father. To her mother's delight, and for reasons unknown to both the patient and her father, Vanessa became dry. Sometime later when she was once more offered milk, she refused it, said she no longer liked it; but she had some ice cream, and once more began to wet the bed, receiving a dressing down from an angry father. In this family milk made one child vomit and a second enuretic; milk did not upset the father but whether it would have upset the mother we may never know, for she hates milk and will never drink it.

There is much circumstantial evidence which suggests that not only allergies in general run in families but that also specific allergies such as asthma and migraine also run in families, and so do specific sensitivities. The more, therefore, that you can identify your own allergies and those of your children, the more you will be able to help each other.

Chapter VIII

INVESTIGATIONS AND MEDICATIONS

P atients with allergies very often expect doctors to give them a battery of skin tests, to tell them all the things they are allergic to, and then to send them home with a prescription for good health. The investigation of allergic problems is never as simple as this.

As you are aware from what you have already read, the story that you have to tell your doctor is of overriding importance, for it provides him with clues that will guide him in his search for the *allergens* that are troubling you. After taking the history and carrying out the physical, your doctor will then probably skin test your child. Skin tests are carried out with specially prepared extracts of house dust, pollens from grasses, weeds, and trees, as well as with extracts of molds, and danders from animals, and with extracts of foods. These extracts are either placed on the skin and a scratch or prick made through them, or they are injected into the skin itself.

The first person to carry out a scratch test was a Dr. Blackley, almost a hundred years ago. He found that when he placed a little of the grass pollen that give him hay fever on the skin of his forearm, and scratched through it, the skin became red, swollen and itchy, and remained so for nearly twenty-four hours. We now know that this reaction occurs when a patient has some of the special ammunition we have called Immunoglobulin E in his armamentarium; this immunoglobulin is attached to special cells in the skin called mast cells.

If the patient is allergic to the substance introduced into his skin, the substance becomes attached to the Immunoglobulin E on the mast cell, and a minor explosion, the positive skin test, occurs. If he is not allergic to the substance, no reaction occurs; the test is negative. When the explosion occurs, histamine is discharged into the tissues. It is histamine that produces the red itchy swelling that is the hallmark of the positive skin test.

But though we know that histamine is set free in the skin by the *allergen,* we do not know for sure that it is this same allergen which is setting histamine free in the nose, lungs, blood vessels, or elsewhere whenever the allergic reaction takes place in the child. If your child's history suggests that his symptoms coincide with the grass pollen season, positive skin tests to grass pollen can be considered confirmatory. If, however, the symptoms are not seasonal, grass pollens cannot be considered the main source of his troubles, though they may be contributory. Skin tests are very helpful in identifying inhalent allergens; they are less helpful in identifying foods.

As we mentioned in the last chapter, some people have sensitized lungs (asthma), some have sensitized blood vessels (migraine), and others sensitized bladders (enuresis). A positive skin test indicates that the allergic reaction is taking place in the skin, but it does not mean, necessarily, that the same allergic reaction is taking place in the lungs, blood vessels, or bladder.

If your child, for example, has asthma and also has a positive skin test to horse dander, but as far as you know, he has never been near a horse and has certainly not been near a horse when he has had an attack of asthma, horse dander may not be causing his asthma. Nevertheless your doctor will ask you to make sure that there is no horse hair in the leather chair in the living room or in the undercarpet, for your son may have been exposed to horse hair in ways that you had not realized.

In some centers patients are now being asked to breathe in the extracts to which they have positive skin tests. In this way it is possible to make sure that these inhalants are actually capable of precipitating attacks of asthma; if they are, they should be avoided.

Scratch tests provide a rough guide, but a more reliable guide is given when the test material is injected into the skin, or as we say, intradermally. These are the intradermal tests. Reactions to *intradermals* tend to be brisker than those to scratches, so weaker solutions are used.

Foods to which your child may be sensitive are best identified by removing them from his diet and waiting to see if his symptoms subside. To be quite certain that the food is to blame, it is necessary to remain off the food for long enough for you to be certain that he is really better. If Jane has a constant *runny nose* and within a week of being placed on a restricted diet her nose clears and the discharge ceases, wait a week and then challenge her with the food that is thought to be causing her symptoms. Be careful to give her plenty of the food, not just a trace. If her cold returns immediately, this would suggest that the food in question is to blame. If you are still not sure, repeat the experiment, just as we did with the little baby who had asthma when she went off the breast and onto the bottle.

If, on the other hand, Jane has headaches or spells of abdominal pain and vomiting which recur every two to four weeks, it will be necessary to keep her off the food (s) for a sufficiently long time, six or eight weeks, for you to be certain that she is or is not better. If she appears to be better, challenge her again with the suspected food (s) , again being sure to give plenty.

If it is thought for one reason or another that a food is causing your child's symptoms, but neither you nor your doctor have any idea which, it will probably be necessary to place her on a very restricted diet, eliminating milk and all dairy products, chocolate, egg, cereals, and certain fruits such as oranges and tomatoes. If her symptoms subside, the foods omitted from the diet may be returned one at a time, not more than one new food being given each week; introduce foods in liberal amounts; any food that causes a return of symptoms should be avoided. Do not add a new food until symptoms caused by the introduction of a previous food have subsided. If your child's symptoms persist, you have either not eliminated the food to which she is allergic, or her symptoms are due to other factors.

According to Dr. Speer, the ten foods in descending order of importance to which people are most commonly allergic are: cow's milk and dairy products, chocolate and cola drinks, corn, citrus fruits, egg, peas and beans, tomato, wheat, apple, cinnamon.

Coloring agents, both in foods as well as in drinks, and medications may also cause trouble. There is sometimes cross-reactivity between closely related foods, so that when citrus fruits are eliminated, oranges, lemons, tangerines, lime, and grapefruit should also be avoided, as well as their juices. Similarly peas, beans, peanut products, and soya should all be eliminated together. When the foods are reintroduced, it may be found that some citrus fruits are tolerated and others not; some people can not take commercial orange juice, it often contains extracts of the peel, but they can take an orange; some people find that the skin of an orange will make their lips blister but that the orange itself does not upset them. The same applies to the various members of the pea family.

The identification of food sensitivities often requires much patience and persistence on the part of both patient and physician. Its success depends in large measure on the experience of the allergist. This being so, ancillary methods are sometimes used. The first is to place suitably diluted drops of food extract under the tongue. This may precipitate symptoms such as headache, a runny nose, or even a cough or wheeze. When this is so, the foods in question should be eliminated from the diet for a trial period, as already indicated, followed by a challenge.

Some allergists prefer to inject food extracts into or under the skin rather than to give them under the tongue, and find that this approach gives the best guide to the food (s) which are causing symptoms. These two ways of trying to determine what a given patient is allergic to are not used by the majority of allergists. To what extent they can be relied on, in both a positive and in a negative way, is not yet certain.

Although avoiding foods helps to eliminate allergies due to these, avoiding inhalants is not always as easy to arrange, and when this is so, the alternatives are either to take medications to control the reactions, or to submit to a series of shots, or a combination of the two. If a series of shots is embarked on, the substance or substances that your child is sensitive to will be given him probably at weekly intervals, but sometimes more frequently. The *shots* sometimes precipitate the symptoms which it is hoped they will eventually relieve; they may aggravate a *runny* nose or wheeze; they may even cause fever. They may also cause a brisk, local reaction in the arm, so that where your child was injected, the arm becomes red and swollen. When this is the case, the *shots* are probably a little too strong and should be weakened, so that they cause no more than a little local reaction. The aim of this form of treatment is to make your child less sensitive to the dust, pollen, or mold that is making him wheeze. It probably does this by stimulating the production of Immunoglobulin G. This type of immunoglobulin ammunition, unlike Immunoglobulin E, usually does not lead to the liberation of histamine when it latches onto the allergen, and because it grasps the allergen while it is still in the blood stream, it is not caught up by Immunoglobulin E, and no histamine is released; no allergic reaction occurs. Unfortunately it may take many months to build up enough Immunoglobulin G to lead to an appreciable relief of symptoms, and shots may need to be continued for several years.

What medications are available? These fall into three main groups, and they are often prescribed in combination.

For an Allergic Rhinitis

Antihistamines are the drugs of most value. These drugs do not prevent the formation of histamine, but when they are present in sufficient quantity, they displace histamine, so that the histamine cannot act on the mucous glands in the nose and bronchial tubes and make them *secrete mucous*. Similarly histamine cannot make the muscles in the bronchial tubes contract, again because the antihistamine is in the way. Unfortunately histamine is not the only substance liberated in the allergic reaction that acts on the bronchi; the other substances are not blocked by antihistamines. So although antihistamines help those who have nasal stuffiness and who make much nasal and bronchial mucous, they do not usually help to control wheezing.

Antihistamines, besides drying secretions in the lungs and nose, tend to make the child drowsy. They are, in fact, good sedatives, some are better sedatives than others. This action is welcome if the drug is taken at night, but it is a nuisance if the drug has to be taken during the daytime, and it can be dangerous if the sufferer plans to or has to drive a car.

Nasal stuffiness can also be reduced by nose drops containing decongestants; these are substances related to epinephrine. They make the small blood vessels contract and so reduce the swelling in the tissues. Some specialists feel that it is unwise to depend too much on *nose drops* of this kind, for their repeated application may eventually harm the lining of the nose.

Asthma

EPINEPHRINE. Those who have had severe attacks of asthma know the great relief that epinephrine can bring. Epinephrine is a normal constituent of the body and is made by the adrenal gland. It is released in greatest amounts in times of stress. It increases the force and action of the heart, it raises the blood sugar, and it increases alertness. In a word, it prepares the individual for action. It also relaxes the bronchial tubes, and it is for this reason that it is given to asthmatics. It makes it possible for the asthmatic to breathe easily again.

Epinephrine, unfortunately, cannot be given by mouth because it is destroyed by the digestive juices, for this reason it must be injected. It is usually injected just under the skin, subcutaneously, great care being taken to avoid a vein. It is such a powerful chemical that if it is given into a vein, it will immediately act on the heart, making it beat violently, so violently that its normal pumping action may be jeopardized. If it is given just under the skin, it reaches the heart and lungs more slowly, and though acting with remarkable rapidity, it does not disturb the heart unduly. A little epinephrine is invaluable, too much can be dangerous. In exceptional cases, such as in severe anaphylactic shock, it may have to be given straight into a vein or even into the heart.

EPHEDRINE. The action of ephedrine is similar to that of epinephrine, but it has the great advantage that it can be given by mouth. It has the disadvantage that its action is slow; epinephrine begins to act within a minute or two of its administration, ephedrine has first to be absorbed; it cannot start acting for 30 to 60 minutes. Besides relaxing the bronchial tubes, ephedrine, unfortunately, also stimulates the heart, making it beat more quickly, and the brain, causing sleeplessness. Asthma is often most troublesome at night, and though the asthmatic usually needs to take his ephedrine at night, he also needs a good sleep. It is therefore customary to give ephedrine at night with a sedative such as phenobarbitone or benadryl.

As a matter of interest ephedrine has been used by the Chinese for 5,000 years; it is obtained from the plant Ma Huang.

ISOPROTERONOL OR ISUPREL. Isoproteronol, like ephedrine, helps the bronchial tubes to relax. It can be given by inhalation, and in fact is usually given this way; it is carried straight down to the lungs and begins to act on the little bronchi, where its action is most needed, almost as quickly as if it had been given by injection. Like epinephrine it is a powerful drug and must not be taken in unlimited amounts, for it can put a strain on the heart by making it beat both rapidly and irregularly.

When this form of treatment, the inhalation of aerosols containing isoproteronol, first became available, it was not realized that severe asthmatics, finding some relief but not sufficient to satisfy their needs, would go on to inhale breath after breath of this medication, but this indeed is what happened. Doctors in England suddenly became aware that there was an increase in the death rate of young adult asthmatics. Deaths from asthma had declined steadily until 1957, when they began to rise. During the next ten years the death rate doubled. Some asthmatics were actually found dead with an inhaler in their hands.

We think, in retrospect, that some of those who died did so because, in an endeavor to relieve their attacks of asthma, they had inhaled and absorbed too much isoproteronol; their hearts had been overstimulated and they had died of an overstrained heart. If your child needs an aerosol containing isoproteronol to help relieve his attacks of asthma, make sure that the amount that he inhales each day is rationed in accordance with your doctor's instructions.

AMINOPHYLLINE. This is a very useful drug which has an action similar to that of ephedrine, though it acts in a different way. It, too, relaxes the bronchial tubes and stimulates the brain and tends to make children wakeful if given at night. It is effective if given by mouth, and because it acts in a different way from ephedrine, it is often given with ephedrine, as the two together seem to be more effective than either alone. One advantage is that it can also be given as a suppository; this is particularly useful

in the treatment of babies and little children who often refuse
to take medicines when they are offered them on a spoon.

The effects of both ephedrine and aminophylline are cumu-
lative; they should therefore never be given more frequently
than is prescribed by your doctor; if you have given your child
one dose and it seems to have helped him and you think a little
more might help, there is a great temptation to repeat the dose
and hope for the best. This can be very dangerous; follow your
doctor's instructions carefully, and when in trouble always contact him.

CORTISONE. When cortisone first became available, it was natural
that it should be given to patients with asthma, for extra cortisone
and closely related substances are made by the body in times of
stress. Asthma itself is a stressful condition, and it was speculated
that additional cortisone might help. It was soon found that this
indeed was the case, and that cortisone helped both the patient
with an acute attack of asthma and also the patient whose day to
day activities were severely curtailed by his asthma. Many such
patients were and still are enabled to lead tolerable, if not completely normal, existences. Cortisone and its derivatives are also
used in the local treatment of eczema.

Many different preparations of cortisone-like substances are on
the market, some being more powerful than others. They are in
constant use, and they have transformed the lives of many asthmatics. Nevertheless we are reluctant to use cortisone* unless we
feel that without it the patient's activities would be severely
limited, for patients who need cortisone become dependent on its
use and are likely to experience certain unfortunate so-called side
effects.

It may make a person put on weight, make his face, neck, body,
and thighs unhealthily fat, and his face red and plethoric. Cortisone, if given for several years, also tends to milk calcium out of
the bones; the bones lose their strength, and the bones in the
spine may even be crushed by the weight they have to carry.
Nerves may be pressed upon, pain may result. Cortisone also
hinders normal growth. This action is of no concern to the adult,

---

* The term cortisone is used to refer both to cortisone and to other cortisone like
substances made by the adrenal glands or given to patients.

but it is of vital importance to the child, for as long as he remains on cortisone, his growth may be hindered or even arrested.

Although it was at first thought that cortisone to be effective had to be given two, three, or four times a day to ensure a constant supply to the tissues, as it is made all the time by the adrenal glands, it has more recently been discovered that in the management of asthma, this is not always the case. Cortisone is often effective if given only once every other day, provided it is given in an appropriate dose. Children and adults when treated in this way often escape unwanted side effects. They do not become too obviously obese nor is their rate of growth unduly retarded.

In concluding this section it should be mentioned that cortisone is normally made by the adrenal glands at a fairly constant rate, depending on the needs of the body; more is made in the morning than in the evening, and more is made in times of stress than in times of tranquility. In the normal course of events a mechanism akin to a thermostat controls the production of cortisone, for when blood levels are low, cortisone production is increased, and when blood levels are high, it falls, just as in the house the furnace is fired when the temperature falls and is extinguished when the temperature rises.

If cortisone is given every day and in large amounts to children, or to adults for that matter, the cortisone thermostat may be turned off altogether, and when the child stops taking cortisone, the body may not start making it again, at least not in amounts necessary to meet stressful situations. It may take several months or a year for the child's adrenal glands to regain their original vitality, and though he may be able to meet his day to day needs, provided these are minimal, he may not be able to meet any additional demands made by stressful situations such as illness, accidents, and operations. He will need extra cortisone at these times. If, when he was given cortisone, it was possible to give it in one *slug* every other day, his thermostat will be less likely to get lazy or rusty, and when cortisone treatment is eventually stopped, his own adrenal glands will usually begin to manufacture it in normal amounts.

DISODIUMCROMOGLYCATE OR INTAL. A few years ago a doctor in England, Dr. Altounyan, who was testing a number of chemicals which he felt might help in the management or treatment of asthma, found that disodiumcromoglycate, though useless in the treatment of an acute attack of asthma, was sometimes little short of miraculous in its prevention. Disodiumcromoglycate, unfortunately, is not absorbed to any appreciable extent if given by mouth, but it is effective if it is inhaled. It is therefore taken as a powder by means of a specially designed inhaler. To be of any value, it has to be inhaled at regular intervals four times a day.

It does not help everyone who has asthma or hay fever, but it helps many. Those who are helped must continue to inhale it, or their allergies will return. They may find so much relief that if they are taking cortisone, they are able to reduce the amount they have to take or even to stop taking it altogether. Disodiumcromoglycate seems to have very few disagreeable side effects; it does not overstimulate the heart or brain, nor does it interfere with growth although it occasionally irritates the bronchial tubes. It is a very valuable addition to the medicine chest of the patient with asthma and hay fever.

Aspirin

We should not close this chapter without a word or two about aspirin. I am sure that all those who read this book will have had at least an occasional aspirin. Some will have taken them on rare occasions, for a toothache for example, others will have taken them more regularly, for headaches, rheumatism, fibrositis and the like. Some will have bought aspirins on their own account over the counter, others will have had them prescribed by doctors, for they are essential for the proper treatment of rheumatic fever and rheumatoid arthritis; they often act like a charm on the feverish child. Aspirins have become essential, if not for life, at least for living. They are nevertheless not free from danger, for a few individuals become sensitive to or intolerant of them. They find that when they take an aspirin they develop a profuse, watery nasal discharge, or they wheeze, or break out in hives. Some patients develop nasal polyps.

Those who are sensitive to aspirin sometimes become sensitive to related compounds such as indomethazin, which is also prescribed for rheumatism, and tartrazine; the latter being a yellow colouring agent often added to medicines. Luckily the aspirin sensitive patient can usually take sodium salicylate, (aspirin is acetyl salicylate), and tylenol. Aspirin sensitivity does not usually develop till middle age, nevertheless if you or your child have respiratory allergies and are taking aspirin, make sure that the aspirin is not compounding your problems.

Chapter IX

APPETITE AND ALLERGIES

I remember as a lad looking forward in the summer to strawberries and cream after cricket, to sausage and mash after football, and to toast with butter and marmalade for breakfast on Sundays (on weekdays we were allowed only butter or marmalade) , and of course, to turkey with all the etceteras on Christmas Day. I still love food; though instead of stuffing myself with goodies—I once adored Cadbury's marshmallow milk chocolate—I now sip a Bristol Milk Sherry or down a dry Martini. There were no foods that I actively hated, and though I naturally preferred tasty to tasteless foods, I thought my parents were reasonable when they made us eat cabbage before apple pie and rice pudding before chocolate. It seemed just and fair to us, for though man cannot live by bread alone, neither can he live only on strawberries and cream.

When I began taking the histories of asthmatic children, I soon learned that children sometimes suffer quite unnecessarily by being made to eat or drink things they actively dislike. One lad, I remember, had been brought up on cod liver oil. Many children were brought up on cod liver oil in England during the war and most loved it. This child did not. But his father insisted on making him take it, for he was a frail lad and prone to chest colds. The vitamin A in cod liver oil was supposed, in the pre-vitamin C era, to protect the respiratory tract against infections. This child fought to avoid his medicine. It was not until he finally succeeded that his respiratory troubles subsided, for he was allergic to cod liver oil.

Another child I remember seeing was pale and underweight and had frequent loose stools; he objected to the eggs, given for their iron content, that his mother gave him. It was not until his mother allowed him to have his own way that his diarrhea cleared and his color improved.

A much older boy was brought to me by his mother as he had lost his appetite and was troubled with frequent spells of abdominal pain. The less he wanted to eat, the more milk his mother gave him. When she was persuaded to let him choose his own menu, he avoided milk and dairy products, ate other foods, and had no more spells of abdominal pain and gained weight.

Whatever the explanation for their problems, these three children would have been spared much illness had they been allowed to eat the foods of their own choosing, or at least to avoid the foods they disliked. These children may have learned, and if so probably unconsciously, that the cod liver oil, egg, and milk made them ill; they may, like the Pavlovian dog, have been conditioned to dislike the foods in question.

But this is not always the case. Some children seem to be born with the distaste for a potentially harmful food. On one occasion my attention was drawn to a four pound baby in the nursery who seemed to be unable to suck and who on this account was losing weight steadily. It was feared that his brain had been damaged, even though his birth had been uncomplicated, and that it was for this reason he *could not suck*. Examination revealed no abnormality. We wondered whether he was not sucking because he did not like his formula, so we offered him breast milk from a bottle. He took it eagerly, sucked greedily, and immediately began to gain weight. A few months later he was given ordinary cow's milk and promptly developed diarrhea. He had to be given a less allergenic formula. He was born with an antipathy to cow's milk, the food which upset him.

I later encountered another baby who was being brought up on the breast and who refused his first feed of formula made from cow's milk. He was thriving on the breast, but the time came when his mother had to go out for the evening. She wanted to make sure that he would take the bottle when it was offered him by their baby-sitter, so she first offered it to him herself. He turned away from the nipple and in every way that a baby can indicated that he would not touch it. But his mother, as so often happens, won the day; she forced a few drops between his lips. He promptly vomited. He was obviously, and subsequent events confirmed this, highly sensitive to milk.

It is characteristic of food-allergic children and adults that they have very capricious appetites, not only disliking certain foods and even refusing them in one form but taking them in another. Many children avoid canned or cooked vegetables, for example, while relishing them raw. I have developed a very healthy respect for a child's likes and dislikes; these can give the doctor a most helpful guide. If your allergic child has a poor appetite, never force him to eat what he would rather avoid.

As allergies run in families, it is not surprising that we should find unexplained likes and dislikes in other members of the family. These are often most striking in the mother; probably, I think, because mothers tend to have more allergies than fathers. It is for this reason that, quite early in our studies, I noted that while the child was drinking milk and being made ill by it, the mother often made a point of avoiding it herself. When I asked the mother why she would not drink milk, she would usually reply that she found the taste unpleasant. She would sometimes say "I hate it."

Many such parents can drink a glass of milk without being upset by it, but others find that if they do so they develop indigestion, nasal stuffiness, or mucous in their throats, symptoms which suggest that they may, like their child, be allergic to milk. Oddly enough this dislike for milk is quite common among women, at least on the North American continent, whether the child is or is not allergic. Twenty per cent of women dislike milk.

A few years ago, when stewardesses served only pop drinks or coffee, milk, and tea, I would ask them whether men and women appeared to be equally fond of milk. "Oh, no," they would reply, "only men drink milk, the women never do." And when asked why this might be so, they would say they thought men preferred milk because so many of them had ulcers, and the women preferred coffee because they considered milk fattening. Whatever the explanation it is certainly a way of life on the North American continent. I have often wondered if this tendency of women to avoid milk may not be one of the reasons why they as a group have fewer heart attacks and less arteriosclerosis than men.

Allergy is full of paradoxes, and while it is true that some people dislike the food to which they appear to be allergic, they sometimes, as I have already mentioned, crave it. Why this should be so, we do not know. Some may crave a food because it brings a temporary relief, much as heroin brings relief to the addict, as though it fulfilled an unmet need. If this is so, there is probably a biochemical or immunological explanation. Some, on the other hand, may have become sensitive to the food because they ate too much of it and sensitized themselves.

If the latter explanation is correct, it would seem wise for the individual who has food allergies to make a point of varying his diet as much as possible and of avoiding overindulgence in any one food. Whatever the explanation once an individual who appeared to crave or be addicted to a food stops taking this food and finds himself relieved of his allergies, he usually has no difficulty in refraining from taking it thereafter.

In addition to their vagaries of appetite, some allergic individuals appear to have a heightened sense of smell. A doctor, who herself has many severe allergies, writes that, "When I am uncomfortable because of my asthma, I am very aware of all kinds of odors which generally are annoying; the smell of food, smell of dust, smell of newspapers, or even stationery." I know of one corn-sensitive and another peanut-sensitive individual whose smell for corn and peanuts respectively is so acute that both automatically detect them long before most people are aware of them. I know a third person with many allergies who is so acutely aware of the smell of gas that she notes gas leaks long before anyone else in the house can detect them.

There comes a time when we should ask ourselves, is it necessary to investigate all allergies? I think the answer to this question at the present time is no. Two of the commonest problems encountered in allergy practice are those of perennial allergic rhinitis in children and adults, and of enuresis. At the present moment we can not always identify the precipitating allergen.

Some individuals with a constant nasal stuffiness, rather than submit to a battery of tests and a series of shots, prefer to use lots of handkerchiefs and an occasional antihistamine; even when they know from experience that house dust bothers them, they still prefer to keep their nice, friendly old carpet in the living room and the house undisturbed; they do not want to radically change their home environment.

Mild allergies of the bladder, for example, that cause an occasional wet bed in a three-year-old can be ignored for the time being in the hopes that the child will, as often happens, grow out of his problem. But if your child's allergies have undesirable side effects, if her constant nasal stuffiness makes her hard of hearing, it should be investigated and treated. Any child who has frequent attacks of bronchitis and asthma deserves study. A child with occasional attacks of tummy pain can, perhaps, be reassured, but the child with severe attacks should be studied; for if the cause can be found and dealt with, he will be spared further attacks of pain and may be spared an unnecessary appendectomy, as well as many incapacitating attacks of migraine in adult life.

If the child has *nervous symptoms,* is always tired, looks pale and has dark circles under his eyes, or if he is hyperactive and drives his parents and teachers up the wall, an attempt should certainly be made to find out why, for if his symptoms are allergic in origin and can be dealt with by the elimination of a few simple foods, the child's future may well be transformed; he will be a better pupil at school and much more popular with his teachers and classmates.

Chapter X

ALLERGIES AND THE AUTONOMIC
NERVOUS SYSTEM

When I go to work in the morning, I first go to the garage, unlock the door, get into my car, start the engine, and when it has warmed sufficiently, let in the clutch and drive off. On the way to the hospital I brake and accelerate, stop and turn as the occasion demands. But whatever is done with the car is done in response to my wishes. It is I who decide how slowly or how swiftly the car will run. The car does nothing on its own account. The same is not true, however, of my body, for though I decide when to get up and when to sit down, when to run and when to walk, the body itself has assumed control of its own really vital functions. My heart beats quickly when I run and slows when I walk or sit down; my sweat glands perspire when my body is warm but not when it is cold; my breathing quickens when I need extra oxygen or have to dispose of extra carbon dioxide but not when I don't. My pupils contract when the light is bright and dilate when it is dark.

These functions are carried out automatically by a series of self-regulating mechanisms. It is just as well that this is so, for had I to consciously regulate my own temperature, heart and respiration rates, I would be fully occupied. I would not have time to attend to other vitally important matters, namely finding the food or fuel my body needs to keep it alive and active; in a primitive society this entails hunting, fishing, and raising crops, in civilized society this entails earning a living.

For reasons that we do not yet fully understand, it is the bodily functions which are normally regulated automatically that are disturbed in the allergic reaction. The asthmatic finds that his breathing is no longer automatically adjusted to meet his needs; he may have to fight for breath, even when he is at rest. He finds, this often happens in the allergic reaction, that he breaks out in a so-called *cold sweat* when he does not need to lose heat. He finds that his stomach, instead of accepting and digesting food, throws it up; his bowels, which should digest and absorb food in a leisurely and efficient manner, hurry it through and he develops diarrhea. He finds that his bladder, which should relax to accommodate urine, cannot do so; it has to be emptied frequently. The heart and blood vessels may also be affected; in anaphylactic shock the blood pressure may fall so low that the pulse becomes quite impalpable. Allergic disorders involve the autonomic nervous system so frequently that we could almost stop talking of allergic diseases and talk instead of diseases of the autonomic system.

There is in the brain a region called the hypothalamus. This is the center which regulates, like a computer or a thermostat, the activities of the autonomic nervous system. We cannot consciously control its activities, but its activities are nevertheless not completely independent of will or emotion, for it has connections with areas concerned both with thought and feeling. It is because of the presence of these connections that problems and worries that exist in our conscious minds can have their repercussions on the hypothalamus and may in this way precipitate asthma, vomiting and diarrhea, profuse sweating, and spells of urgency and frequency of micturition.

Because the autonomic nervous system controls and the allergic reactions may involve identical body systems, it is sometimes difficult to decide whether it is an emotional disturbance or whether it is an allergic reaction which is responsible for the patient's symptoms. This is understandable, for asthma can make a person frightened, just as in some allergic people fright can bring on an attack of asthma. Worry can cause diarrhea, while diarrhea, particularly if it has no obvious explanation, naturally causes worry.

From what I have told you, it must be apparent that though we know a great deal about the manifestations and management of allergic problems and though we know much more than we did a few years ago about the mechanisms underlying the allergic response, there is much still to be learned. Allergy is full of unsolved problems and unanswered questions. Why did Jimmy appear to be born with asthma? Why was his brother symptom free as a baby and only developed asthma when he was six? Why do oranges give Janice eczema, make Jim wet the bed at night, and give his mother migraine? Why does house dust give Brent a stuffy nose and yet make his sister wheeze? Why do some people outgrow their allergies while others seem to accumulate more and more?

There are answers to all these questions, but they will be slow in coming unless those with allergic problems start to channel their resources not only into the provision of help for allergic individuals but also into establishing, supporting, and developing research in the field of allergy.